LOOKING UP

LOOKING UP

The Complete Guide to Looking and Feeling Good for the Recovering Cancer Patient

SUZY KALTER

MEDICAL DIRECTORS
Steven P. Kalter, M.D.
and
Debra C. Kalter, M.D.

Photographs by Harry Langdon

McGRAW-HILL BOOK COMPANY

New York St. Louis San Francisco Bogotá Hamburg Madrid Mexico
Milan Montreal Panama Paris São Paulo Tokyo Toronto

PLEASE NOTE

The author is not a medical doctor and does not directly or indirectly dispense medical advice for the treatment of cancer or intend in any way to diagnose or prescribe. The intent of this book is to offer beauty and fitness advice to cancer patients, specifically those undergoing radiotherapy and chemotherapy. Please check with your doctor and oncological nurse regarding your specific case vis-à-vis any recommendations offered in this text. While the conditions described in these pages are accurate, they represent the widest range of possibilities. It is possible that you will experience none of the side effects mentioned; it is improbable that all of them will affect you. Your doctor probably knows everything in this book; it is unlikely he will tell you about it unless you ask specifically.

1 2 3 4 5 6 7 8 9 DOC DOC 8 9 8 7

ISBN 0-07-033252-5

Library of Congress Cataloging-in-Publication Data

Kalter, Suzy.
   Looking up.

   1. Cancer—Patients—Rehabilitation.   2. Beauty, Personal.   3. Cancer—Treatment—Complications and sequelae.   I. Title.
RC262.K354   1987   616.99'406   87-4164
ISBN 0-07-033252-5

Book Design by Kathryn Parise

to
GLORIA VERSTEIN KALTER
1925–1981

Mammograms can be wrong.

MEDICAL CONSULTANTS

William Fein, M.D.

Robert J. Futeran, M.D.

Debra C. Kalter, M.D.

Seymour S. Kalter, Ph.D.

Steven P. Kalter, M.D.

Arnold W. Klein, M.D.

Herbert Rappoport, M.D.

Lon Smith, M.D.

MODELS

The Laughing Women

Barbara Cady

Giovanna Gentili

Sharon Torres

Judith Evans Thomas

Patty Franklin

Marianne Gray

Julie Fox

Joan Paul

Makeovers

Sharon Torres

Jane Shimizu

Karen Luce

Geri Connor

Contents

Foreword   xv

Preface   xvii

Acknowledgments   xix

Chapter One / *LOOKING GOOD IS THE BEST REVENGE*   3

Why Me?   3

The Healing Art of Looking Good   5

Baseline Beauty Checkup   7

Present-Day Cancer Treatment   9

    Chemotherapy   9

    Radiotherapy   10

    Immunotherapy   11

    Interferon   12

State of Readiness   12

Chapter Two / *HAIR CARE*   15

The Rapunzel Syndrome   15

Drugs, Toxins, and Their Effects on Hair   18

Before Chemotherapy   20

Fallout   24

The Emperor's New Hair   25

Acceptable Losses   26

The Crew Cut   28

Types of Hair Loss   29

Preventing Hair Loss   31

Now What?   33

Chapter Three / WIGS AND WITHOUT   37

To Wig or Not To Wig   37

Wig Tricks   38

Wigging Up   40

   The Custom-Made Wig   45

   The Ready-to-Wear Wig   46

Wig Rip-offs   48

   Hairpieces   49

Thin-Hair Tricks   50

The Beginner's Wig   51

Wigs and Styles   54

Other Wigs   55

How to Choose a Wig   57

Wig Styling   59

Wig Care   60

Wig Supplies   61

Wigless Possibilities   61

Bald Is Beautiful   62

Covered Heads   63

Hat Tricks   73

Growing In   74

Does She or Doesn't She?   75

Perms   77

Virgin Hair   77

Private Matters   78

Chapter Four / *SKIN AND MAKEUP*   81

Skin Facts   81

The Effects of Treatment   83

   Dry Skin   85

   Rashes and Red Skin   87

   Hyperpigmentation   87

   Phototoxicity   88

Temporary Damage versus Permanent Damage   89

Radiant Irradiated Skin   89

Scars: Camouflage and Treatment   90

Skin Cancers   92

   Malignant Melanoma   93

Sun Care   95

Makeup   95

   Inpatient Makeup   96

   Outpatient Makeup   98

The Two-Minute Face   103

The Two-Second Blush   105

Makeovers   105

   Sharon Torres   107

   Jane Shimizu   107

   Karen Luce   109

   Geraldine Connor   111

You in Transition   113

Chapter Five / BODY TALK   115

Eyes   115

   Visible Differences   115

   Eye Problems   116

Eyebrows and Eyelashes   119

   Eyebrows   120

   Eyelashes   121

   Eye Tricks   125

Lungs   126

Head and Neck   127

Hands and Nails   128

   Hands   128

   Nails   129

Feet   134

   Toenails   134

Teeth, Mouth, and Lips   136

   Teeth   136

Mouth   138

Lips   141

Smoking   142

Drinking   142

Oral Cancer   142

Chapter Six / PRIVATE TALK   145

The Unspeakable   145

Breasts—Fear and More Fear   146

   Breast Facts   147

   Breast Cancer   148

   Treatments   148

   Recovery   152

   The New You   156

   Breast Tricks   157

   Buying a Breast   159

   Reconstruction   162

   Immediate Gratification   164

   The Waiting Game   165

   Nipples   166

   Preventive Mastectomy   167

Ostomies   167

   Caring for an Ostomy   169

Gynecologic Matters   170

   "Plumbing"   170

Chapter Seven / DIET AND EXERCISE   173

   Figure Control   173

   Mini-Meals   177

   Mother Was Right   178

   Food Aversions   178

   Vitamins   179

   Calorie Counting   180

   Bloating   180

   Soft and Simple   181

   Exercise   183

   Postmastectomy Exercises—Beginner   185

   Postmastectomy Exercises—Intermediate (with
   Weights)   200

   Leg Exercises   210

Chapter Eight / FEELING GOOD   215

   Feelings   215

   Periods of Adjustment   217

   Members of the Club   218

   Coping Strategies—A Hero Is More Than a
   Sandwich   219

   Information Please   220

   Talking It Out   223

   Support Systems   224

   The Buddy System   225

Taking Responsibility 226

Positive Denial 227

Antidepression Treatment 228

Religion 230

Getting Better 230

Makeup Shopping List 232

Personal Resource List and Phone Numbers 233

Ask Your Doctor 234

Resource List 235

Cancer Information Service 235

Support and Information Groups 236

Beauty Supplies 237

Turbans 237

Wigs 237

Patient Diary 239

Index 243

Foreword

Beauty is an arresting quality that has foresight. Every woman can create an illusion of beauty which may be more arresting and certainly more enduring through the years than that which nature bestows so bountifully on the young.

There are many effective techniques in cosmetic science that we can and should use to enhance the facade. But the important foundation does come from within, thereby making the use of these deft touches effective, and thus true beauty is enhanced with the years and is a joy forever.

The cancer patient is no different. The patient who looks her best and feels her best is the patient who has done something to help herself to recovery. There has never been a more important time for a woman to give herself some special care, to take a little extra time for herself and her looks.

For years I have treated women with cosmetics and skin care the world over in my many salons. I have noticed that of the thousands of women who come to me for advice and care, most come for what they consider the special occasions of their lives—a wedding, a special birthday, a public appearance, an important date, a gala ball. Very few come in when they are ill or under stress. Yet this is the time a woman most needs a helping hand. This is one of those special times that beauty care can offer very special benefits. If you are being treated for cancer, it is a very special time in your life and it should be treated as such.

I have worked together with cancer patients and doctors. I am keenly aware of the physical and emotional ravages of cancer and cancer care. Yet no one knows more than I, and perhaps Ms. Kalter, the benefits of cosmetologic care at a time like this. I firmly believe that if you look good, you feel good. Even if you can't look your very best, you *can* look better. If you look better, you *feel* better.

It's also a matter of self-esteem. If you look good and you like your-self in the mirror, then you like the people around you. You give peo-ple a chance to help you and you meet them much more than half way. You are ready to face the challenges of the modern cancer patient.

Today's cancer patient has much to look forward to. The immediate period of diagnosis, surgery, and treatment is a strenuous one, but one copes and gets through it. While you are coping, you must deal with two different problems that will affect your looks: the cancer and the chemotherapy. The knowing patient understands that these are two separate matters. She isolates them in her mind. Rather than feeling overwhelmed by the combination, she sees them as a dynamic duo—part of a chain reaction that will lead to good health. The chemotherapy will knock out the cancer; together they both will pass from her body and she will be restored to a healthful state. The immediate problems are transient ones. Many of them will go away. Some of them will create new realities that are difficult at first but are accepted and as-similated into the lifestyle. For the time being, you need only cope. And the best way to cope is to pay attention to your looks; to reach out not only for medical help but for cosmetical help.

There is no magic that can be offered to you. There are no beauty secrets that will transform you overnight. However, there *are* certain cosmetological truths. This book helps spell them out.

I have read this book and suggest it as must reading to every woman, whether she is a patient or not. What this book teaches you is the most essential lesson of all—you can always make yourself feel better by doing something about your appearance. This book does more than answer the questions that cancer patients ask. It provides hope. It is a friend at a time when too few women know to reach out—to each other, to a product, to a mirror, to a lipstick. Reach and receive. You will feel the better for it.

Aida Grey
Beverly Hills

Preface

I first began this book over ten years ago. As my family began to deal with my mother's cancer diagnosis and her subsequent treatment, I realized there was a definite need for a book that told all. Jane Brody, of the *New York Times,* had just gone through the same experiences with her mother. She also knew the value of a book about cancer.

When her book was published, it was considered a wild and daring feat—a breakthrough in publishing. Until then, no major publisher would go near the subject of cancer. Having just published Brody's book, the industry felt it had done its good deed and that there was no possible market for another cancer book—especially a beauty book.

As I worked with my mother and her illness, I continued to see a need for this book. My mother lost all of her hair three separate times. She gracefully hid pieces of life-sustaining equipment under her clothes. She covered her brown spots with camouflage. Throughout it all, she took notes.

This book grew from my original outline, my mother's and my notes during her illness, and new research and interviews done after the book was finally sold. It took Joan Stewart a year and a half of unrelenting work to find a major publisher who would take the risk of printing a beauty book for cancer patients.

This book is not really a book about cancer. It is a book about the cosmetic effects of chemotherapy and radiotherapy. While it is mainly intended for cancer patients, parts of it will also be helpful to alopecia patients and burn victims. It is not a book of frothy promises or vigorous hand-holding. I cannot tell you that everything's going to be all right, that you will live forever. I cannot even assure you that after treatment you will look and feel exactly the same as before.

I can tell you that, with expertise, there is a good chance you will look the same after treatment. Maybe even better. I can also tell you that it doesn't really matter. What matters is that you look and feel the very best you can under any given set of circumstances—that you do not become depressed, waste away, or go into hiding—from your friends, your family, or yourself.

This book is a compilation of information gleaned from doctors, nurses, medical journals, and interviews with patients. It is also Gloria Kalter's legacy. Each woman accepts and rejects various things from her own mother. What you will read is everything my mother taught me.

Acknowledgments

This book was made possible by the dedication of my friends and family who hung in there with me, first to convince a publisher to take on this book and then while I worked without income for a year. It was a very difficult year.

I can't thank my agent, Joan Stewart, enough for her faith in me, my book, and my mother. Her assistant, Cherise Wolas, was wonderful on follow-through and hand-holding—thank you.

Tom Miller, my editor, bought the book with loving care and has given it special nourishment and attention in memory of his mother, Anna Gertrude Holmes Miller.

This has, above all, been a family project. My brother and sister, Dr. Steven P. Kalter and Dr. Debra C. Kalter, worked as medical directors of the project and pored over the manuscript. My father, Dr. S. S. Kalter, also worked on the manuscript, and never yelled at me once. My sister-in-law, Karen, became the first family member to use the book. My husband Michael Gershman and our son Aaron suffered not only the usual insults of an author hard at work but the additional burden of a bald wife and mother. I thank them for their patience and understanding, and I'm sorry you didn't like my wig, Mike.

Our adopted family, the Feins, also played a substantial role in producing this book. There probably would not have been a book at all without the help of Dr. William Fein, whose enthusiasm for the project became tangible support in a myriad of ways. Stephanie Fein assisted at the photography sessions.

Harry Langdon, Trisha Burlingham, and all the Langdon staff were dedicated to the project from the beginning and have earned a special place in my heart with their hard work; thanks also to the other members of the photography team: Mary Davenport of Eva Gabor International, Josef Scigliano and Marguerite White of Eva Gabor International, Sachi of Michaeljohn, Mark Sennet, who came through true-blue (yet again) and photographed the "Suzy Bald" series from the minute my hair hit the linoleum to when it became "socially acceptable." I thank him with hugs and kisses and fondly remember his father, Chester Sennet.

I also got a lot of help with wigs from this country's leading experts. Many thanks to Eva Gabor, Gloria Luckinbill at Rogers & Cowan, Audrey Cohen, René of René of Paris, Tomi Calhoun and Chuck Reese at Wigs of France, Bob Akre of A Gentleman's Choice in Hollywood, California, and Brenda Kay at Ladies Image in Portland, Oregon.

Numerous doctors and health experts helped with this book, of course. The medical consultants are listed separately, but I would especially like to thank Ellen Waiseman of the Breast Center in Van Nuys, California, for her time and phone calls on behalf of this book; Dr. Herb Rappoport became an instant friend and helped recruit models for me from his practice. The UCLA Medical Library and the Yale–New Haven Hospital Library provided much of the research material.

Also, several very good friends of mine underwent chemotherapy while I was writing this book—Rudi Gernreich, Marcia Vickery Wallace, and Estelle Endler. Their input is woven into the text, as is the help given me by Paul Baumrind and the many other patients who answered questionnaires and allowed me to interview them.

Barbara Cady, my good friend and a double survivor, is the main model used in the book; I thank her for her time, her help, and many years of loyal friendship and chicken dinners, as I thank all the models in this book—survivors all. I must especially thank Karen Luce for appearing in these pages. Ms. Luce is not a cancer patient but suffers from alopecia universalis and is spokeswoman for Help Alopecia International Research (HAIR). I could not find a totally bald cancer patient (including no eyebrows and eyelashes) who was willing to be photographed "naked." Karen came to the rescue, because we both thought it was desperately important for this state of grace to be represented in the book. Thank you for your courage, Karen—and everyone.

Although William Safire of the *New York Times* has assured me that "he" is the universal pronoun, I have taken the liberty of labeling all patients in this book as "she" and all doctors as "he." This does not mean that the information in this book is not valid for male patients or that there are no women doctors—it is merely a means of simplification. Hope that's okay, Bill!

LOOKING UP

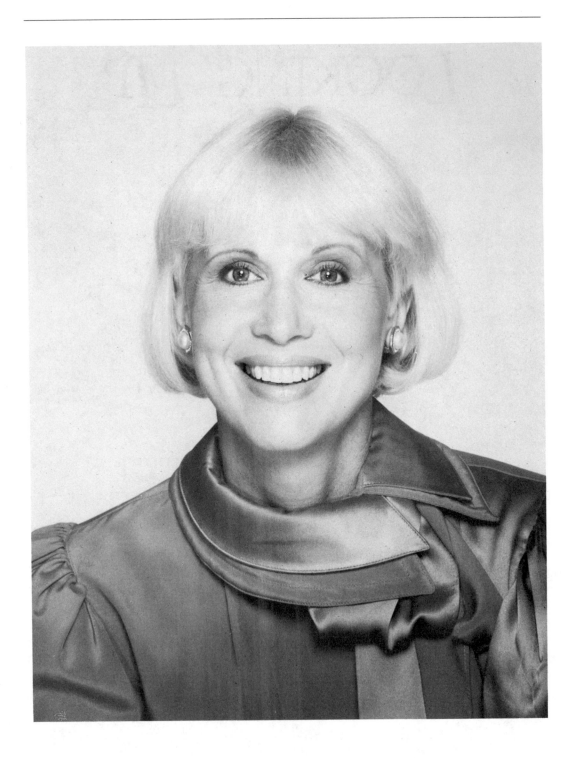

Chapter One

LOOKING GOOD *IS* THE BEST REVENGE

Why Me?

Every cancer patient in the world asks herself one and only one important question—"Why me?" There is no real answer to that question.

For some, the answer is only slightly more apparent; smokers do get lung cancer more frequently than nonsmokers; some cancers run in families; there are environmental factors known to cause cancer.

But even for those who have some clues, the deeper question still cries out to be answered, *"Why me?"* Why not the person across the street? In the next office? In another family? Of all the millions of people in the world—Why me?"

And still there is no answer. There is only a comeback.

After the shock, after the immediate anger, after the hurt; when the part of you that has been screaming out "Why me?" can answer back with a far more powerful question, "Why *not* me?" After the tears and the whispers and the burning lies, you are left with only one truth: You cannot change the facts. You *can* change the way you deal with them.

As a cancer patient, not only is looking good the best revenge, it is one of the best medical breakthroughs you can make for yourself. If you want to lie back and cry and moan and bathe in self-pity, you are welcome to do so. If you're ready to fight, you can start now.

It is only human to ask "Why me?" but for the people who are ready to accept that such a question can never be sufficiently answered, the next most human reaction is to ask to survive. It is only human to feel cheated, abandoned, and bereft of courage. But given the choice, you have no choice. You choose life.

You are about to enter a world where you will have very little control over your body. But you do have control over your mind and your heart. You'll need both now to get you through this—to help you survive. They can set you free to do the important work you now have to do—the work of surviving.

Your medical team can do miraculous things for you. But you are not powerless. Nor are you alone.

Cancer is not an automatic death sentence. The growing population of cancer survivors is changing the face of medicine. Advances are made on a weekly basis, with different results for different forms of cancer. There are multiple types of cancers; there are hundreds of thousands of patients who are responding well to modern treatments. Many of them will live out their natural life span. For more and more people, radiotherapy and chemotherapy will be remembered as a necessary inconvenience in the game of life.

This book is for the woman who knows that she alone cannot cure herself of cancer, but that she can put on lipstick, spruce up her face, and put up one hell of a fight. Hope is no longer a thing with feathers. Hope is the realization that you have it within you to fight back—to screw your courage to the sticking point and then smile your most radiant smile.

Eva Gabor was at her beauty parlor one day when she saw a famous actress who had a serious disease and was commonly known to be seriously ill and not far from death. Nonetheless, the woman kept her weekly hair appointment. "How are you?" Eva asked her one day.

"I've never been better, thank you," replied the grande dame with a glowing smile.

She was lying, of course. But if you whistle a happy tune, sometimes you can fool yourself as well.

The essence of the fight comes from the knowledge that beauty is more than skin deep. Wanting to survive may not be enough in the final analysis, but it will get you a long, long way. Hope is the basis of your tomorrow.

The Healing Art of Looking Good

Two valuable pieces of information of a nonmedical nature have recently made themselves known to doctors and patients alike:

- Laughter cures.

- Looking good counts a lot too.

That's not to say that entering a hospital for treatment of a life-threatening disease is a joking matter or a beauty contest. But patients who manage to find, or keep, their sense of humor and who have enough self-esteem to care about what they look like have a healing edge on patients who do not.

The psychology of looking good is a relatively new one. The women's movement had most of us convinced that looking good was a vanity attached to the wrong sensibilities—that women were trained to look good because they traded openly on the market with their sexuality and their looks. Yet psychologists who study attractiveness have discovered that looking good is actually money in the bank, a better job, and a stronger position in society. It is also a strong indicator of mental attitude.

In a study at Scripps College in Claremont, California, two psychologists found that the more attractive a person makes him- or herself, the more likely it is that people remember what he or she says. "The more attractive a person appears," stated the study, "the more accurately viewers—both male and female—remembered what was said. If you want your words to make a lasting impression, it's important to be concerned about appearance. This is true not only in first meetings but any time you want to get your message across."

In a study at the University of Pennsylvania, women aged 60 and over were divided into two groups. One group was given makeovers, free cosmetics, and helpful hints on appearance by professionals from Elizabeth Arden: The other group—the control group—did not get makeup and received no training or encouragement in the field of beauty; they were merely asked to sort cosmetics by color preference as part of what they were told was a different study. When asked a series of questions about their psychological well-being, the women who had received the cosmetic education revealed themselves to be much happier than the women in the control group. Their make-overs had not only "enhanced their appearance and self-esteem but rekindled their desire to socialize with others."

In a recent study at a psychiatric hospital, Mary Kay Cosmetics experts elicited the first response from a woman who had not spoken or smiled in years. She was made up three different times. After the third time, to the astonishment of her medical team, she actually smiled.

Thomas F. Cash, a psychology professor at Old Dominion University in Norfolk, Virginia, wrote a paper for the *Journal of Cosmetics, Toiletry and Fragrance Association* that posited that a cultural bias has prevented us from exploring the obvious benefits of looking good because we like to think we are above judging a person by his or her looks. For years we have been denying the connection, says Cash.

With the new acceptance that makeup acts as a psychological lift comes the acceptance that makeup can benefit a patient in many ways. Wearing makeup undoubtedly makes you look better; looking better *does* make you feel better. People who feel better show more self-confidence and higher self-esteem, which helps you deal with the world in a more positive manner. A positive attitude affects the people around you and reflects back again—everyone responds better to a well-groomed person. While cosmetic therapy has not yet become common in this country, doctors in several other countries, such as Great Britain, Australia, New Zealand, and Japan, have considered it a vital part of cancer treatment since the 1950s.

In the United States there is a new specialty among makeup artists— paramedical cosmetology. Marvin Westmore, scion of the famous Hollywood Westmore family, has transformed many an actor into a lizard and many a patient into a prettier, more comfortable human being. He often works with plastic surgeons, but considers it his job to teach patients how to use makeup to create "the ultimate illusion." Many of his patients have congenital defects; many are children who are able to hide their problems with cosmetics. The field is a new one. Medical insurance does not yet cover the expenses incurred, yet the movement is obvious and welcome. Makeup and medicine are just beginning to merge. Within the next decade, cosmetic treatment in hospitals will be part of the regular program of recovery.

"The effort to put on makeup and attempt to look better is a reflection of healthy self-respect," says Dr. Elizabeth L. Auchincloss of Payne Whitney Psychiatric Clinic in New York.

So pull your self-respect out of the drawer and send out for a bottle of perfume. Make or buy some audio cassettes for your headset—you'll want a nice selection of material that makes you laugh: Don Rickles, Joan Rivers, whoever you like best. Your body may have been invaded by an unwanted foreigner, but this is not something you need to take lying down.

The fight has just begun.

Baseline Beauty Checkup

Before you begin treatment, and as you adjust to the changes that are now a part of your new life, you should take some time to fill in a Baseline Beauty Profile. This is not a frivolous exercise and will provide information important to you, your nurse, and your doctor as your treatment progresses. Get a family member or intimate friend to help you, if you need some help, but do attempt to record your current condition at the time of diagnosis. There are diary pages in the back of this book that you may want to use as you proceed with your treatment. These pages will prompt you to get out your most secret feelings and will also keep track of your ups and downs, mentally and physically, as you begin your fight. They will also serve as the kind of medical record that no doctor can keep for you, because you, more easily than he, will notice changes in your body that need to be reported. Being aware of what's happening to your body is one of the most effective ways to beat cancer.

It's important that you be as honest as possible in your Baseline Beauty Profile and in your diary notes. Both are tools to help you; they need never be shown to anyone.

Beauty and good health are intertwined. Getting a good picture of what you look like now, before you begin chemotherapy, will help you measure your progress as you begin the business of surviving.

Baseline Beauty Profile

Name: _____   Date of diagnosis: _____

Date: _____   Type of cancer: _____

HAIR

My hair color is (attach sample of hair with tape):

My hair is colored with (name of product and color name and/or number):

The texture of my hair is:

My hair is (circle one):   thick   thin   average

MOUTH

Check the inside of your mouth for sores and color. Mouth and tongue should be an even shade of pink—if pink, write pink. If red, white, or blotchy—report it. Report any abnormalities in this space. Note any stains or discolorations that may now exist on your teeth.

SKIN

Note any moles, rashes, discolorations, or pigmentary markings that you have currently. Check for changes in skin regularly during chemotherapy and radiation treatment and report them to your doctor. Take stock of your moles and birthmarks every six months unless you are a melanoma patient—in which case take stock every two to three months.

FITNESS

Rate your fitness and give a brief description of your everyday physical activities. If you work out regularly, explain your exercise program.

Present-Day Cancer Treatment

There are many, many forms of cancer and several different methods of treating it. Treatment varies most importantly from patient to patient but also from doctor to doctor, hospital to hospital. New drugs and methods of treatment are being tried constantly; experimental work is being done all over the world. It is impossible, and impractical, to compare your treatment to anyone else's. Yet despite the differences in each case, many people react more or less the same way when they are treated with certain techniques.

Chemotherapy

Nicknamed "chemo," *chemotherapy* is a shortened term for "chemical therapy." Chemotherapy was first used against cancer in the 1940s and has become more and more sophisticated since then. The basic principle behind it is simple and increasingly effective: if cancer cells can, by chemical means, be killed or prevented from dividing and spreading, the patient will survive her illness. Because, at this time, there is no way to target just the malignant cells, chemical treatment affects all cells of the body—causing the side effects so many people know and fear.

Chemotherapy can be administered in numerous ways:

- By mouth (not frequent)

- Intramuscularly (unusual)

- Intravenously (most common)

- By indwelling catheters or subclavian lines (becoming increasingly popular)

Subclavian lines are a variation on the intravenous theme. Another variation is the use of an infusion pump (Harvard pump), which provides a steady low dose of medication, is portable (it's usually strapped to the body or hooked onto a belt), and often minimizes the side effects caused by higher doses of monthly chemo treatments.

The most common cosmetic side effects of chemotherapy are hair loss, mouth sores, and changes in nails and skin. Few patients have lasting side effects from treatment, although that varies with the type of drug and dosage required.

Radiotherapy

Radiotherapy is radiation treatment. Radiotherapy is actually now divided into two schools, "old" and "new." The "old" has been around since the 1920s and has been quite successful. The theory behind radiotherapy is essentially the same as for chemotherapy—the cancer cells are killed and prevented from multiplying and dividing by the use of x-rays. While chemotherapy is carried by the blood and does its work throughout the body, radiotherapy is focused on a specific area. Some healthy cells are killed during the irradiation process.

Radiation therapy may be external or internal. In internal treatments, an isotope (in this case, a radioactive element) is placed in the body in an existing or surgically created cavity or is implanted in the body with some access outside of the body. For example, radioactive rods can be implanted in a breast—they are inserted from the outside, fitted under the skin, and then secured outside the skin a few inches away from the point of entry. External treatments include a variety of methods and the use of some new, exciting machinery.

Radiation may be used as a possible cure for cancer, to reduce the size of a tumor before surgery (called *debulking*) or to bring relief from pain (called *palliation*). It is often used in conjunction with other treatments, such as chemotherapy.

Hyperthermia, a recently developed form of radiotherapy, involves bringing the body temperature to a level high enough to kill off the invading cancer cells and is used in conjunction with chemotherapy or traditional radiotherapy. Usually the tumor is first irradiated; then the patient undergoes heat treatments in which her body temperature is raised to approximately 104°F. The temperature of the tumor is brought to 110 to 114°F. There are several methods of applying the technique—some done under general anesthesia, some done with microwaves. So far, tumors close to the surface of the skin have yielded better results than ones buried deep within the body or tucked under vital organs. The process is still considered highly experimental; there are a growing number of radiotherapists who now specialize in hyperthermia.

Another new variation of radiotherapy that is in the experimental stages is *photoradiation*, which is being tested on skin cancers, as well as on stomach, esophageal, and bladder cancers. Doctors use a red laser light and a drug called *HPD*. The patient is first injected with the drug and then exposed to a red light within seventy-two to ninety-six hours. The combination of the light and the drug works to shrink or dissolve a tumor. Often a tumor that has been considered inoperable can be treated with photoradiation and then removed surgically.

Cosmetic side effects from radiotherapy include possible hair loss and changes in skin color or pigmentation.

Immunotherapy

Immunotherapy is still largely experimental. It works on the premise that something in the body's own immune system can be triggered to do what the body's immune system has always done best—fight off disease. Many scientists believe that cancers get their start in life because something has gone haywire in the patient's body in the first place; that her immune system, which is supposed to fight off invaders, has somehow failed to get cracking on the cancer cells. Doctors are using immunotherapy to fight fire with fire.

There are many different approaches to immunotherapy, and new ones are being developed daily. The most common technique is called *nonspecific immunotherapy*; the intent is to stimulate the patient's immune system to fight back by introducing a bacterial extract that will hopefully rally the antibodies for an attack. The most widely used bacteria for this is *bacillus Calmette-Guérin* (BCG). BCG has already been tried and discontinued on patients with melanoma or breast cancer. It is still being used, however, for superficial bladder cancer.

Active immunotherapy uses some of the cellular material from the patient's own tumor, with the hope that this will stimulate the immune system to form specific antibodies to fight the already existing cancer cells.

Passive immunotherapy involves the injection of antibodies from a healthy donor, the idea being that the donor's antibodies will be strong enough to take over and attack the invading cancer.

At this time, immunotherapy is used only in conjunction with other treatments.

The use of *monoclonal antibodies* is another very new type of immunotherapy that has the promise to become a medical miracle. Referred to in lay language as "magic bullets," monoclonal antibodies are aimed at certain sites in the body in order to do very specific work. They are currently used in laboratory tests, both to locate tumors and to bring drugs to a certain place inside the body where they can do their work just on the tumor and not on healthy parts. In clinical testing, monoclonal antibodies are being used on some lymphoma and leukemia patients.

Interferon

Interferon is not one treatment but several—there are three types of interferons. An interferon is a class of proteins that induces noninfected cells to attack the bad guys and prohibit the spread of disease when the body is invaded by a virus. Naturally this sounds like a great way to fight cancer. The major problem so far has been the manufacture of interferons, since they are made by the human body and only in small quantities. There has been some recent success with synthetic interferons and several cases of cancer patients who claim to be alive today because of the treatment.

There are no specific cosmetic side effects, although fatigue is widely reported.

State of Readiness

Whatever form of treatment, or combination of treatments, you are receiving—or are about to receive—doctors and nurses note one very important ingredient that is not chemical. It's known as the patient's *state of readiness for change.*

Each person deals with her diagnosis in her own way. Some patients will deny that they are ill; some patients will accept that they are ill and decide to fight back with a vengeance.

It is possible for a person to go from diagnosis to cure without ever coming to grips with her disease. However, health experts have found that the patient who recovers faster and has fewer side effects during treatment is the one who has learned to accept the diagnosis, who wants to be informed and involved, who is in a state of readiness for change and has therefore accepted the fact that life is going to be different for a while.

How well you cope with the realities of a mastectomy, an ostomy, or a hair loss mostly depends on your state of readiness and ability to be flexible.

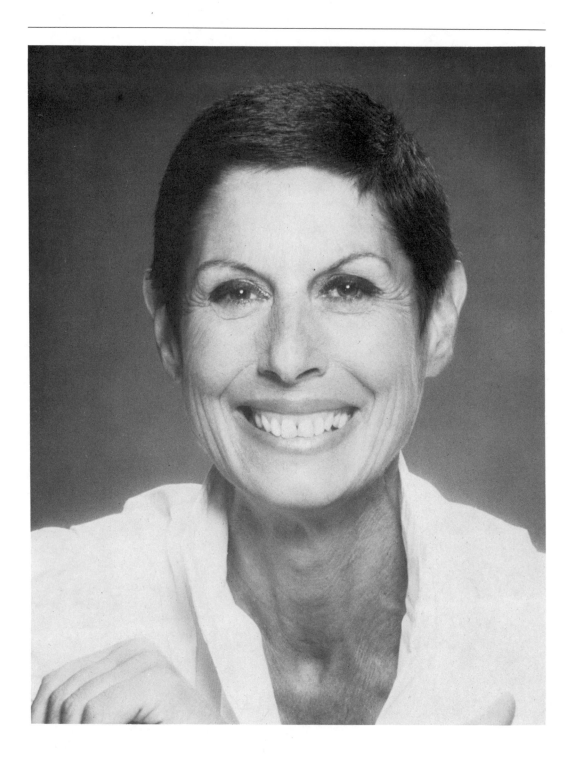

Chapter Two

HAIR CARE

The Rapunzel Syndrome

You remember Rapunzel. "Rapunzel, Rapunzel, let down your hair," shouted the prince, and good old Rapunzel tossed her golden mane out the tower window and let the prince clamber his way to the top.

Now, we have to give Rapunzel and her lover a lot of credit for ingenuity. We won't even think about the practical aspects of the feat, since that could destroy the fantasy. Let's get to the root of the matter—Rapunzel, bless her generous little heart, was the first victim of the Rapunzel syndrome. She took her hair for granted.

Ask a modern woman what her favorite part of her body is, and she will name a part of her anatomy or tell you her least favorite part of her anatomy. She too suffers from the Rapunzel syndrome—she doesn't even *know* how much of her "look" is dependent on her hair. In fact, she takes her hair so much for granted that she only realizes its importance to her when she faces the possibility of losing it.

Few women are unfamiliar with the havoc that can be wreaked on their lives when they feel their hair is out of control; or worse, in control of them. Yet few of them count their blessings that they have hair at all.

For most of us, how our hair looks directly affects how we feel—in terms of both our mood and our feelings of self-worth. This applies to men as well as to women and accounts for the man who parts his hair on the far side to cover a partially balding pate. Such a man is hiding from the world not a scalp, but a piece of his own vulnerability. We're all very quick to complain about our hair, but not so quick to appreciate the fact that we have it at all. Until we might not have it any more.

Organized religion has long recognized the fact that hair is one of life's most sturdy vanities. The Bible advises that, on her wedding day, the bride should prepare herself for the big event with a ritual bath that includes a haircut. Traditionally, hair was cropped short and the bride was presented with a *sheital*—a preformed wig—which she would wear for the rest of her life. The sheital served to separate the women from the girls, so that men could tell at a glance who was available and who was not. Natural hair was considered a sexual lure. Girls were allowed this vanity, while married women, for obvious reasons, were not. Married women were supposed to be unattractive to other men; at the same time, because a woman without hair wasn't too attractive, she wasn't likely to fool around or even think juicy thoughts. Of course, a husband who loved his wife would think she was beautiful no matter how much hair she had, so everyone lived happily ever after.

Nuns of many orders have also been asked to give up their hair, but not for sexual reasons. The church well understood the cosmetic value of hair. Women who were asked to give up the outside world and its adornments were asked to forfeit their hair as they did all objects of vanity. In the world of God, hair is unimportant. The novitiate who is unwilling to part with her hair still has some serious questions about the world she is being asked to give up.

For the secular world, hair has held various meanings, both social and political. In Victorian times, a girl became a woman on her sixteenth birthday, when she was allowed to wear her hair up—thus proclaiming her availability in the marriage market. As a new age began after World War I, women had their hair bobbed to show their freedom. Although the musical *Hair* was actually about the war in Vietnam, the length and unruliness of the antihero's hair stood for every ounce of rebellion within him, serving as the ultimate antiestablishment statement. The mandatory cutting of one's hair—especially to the army regulation length at the time of basic training—was considered an infringement of personal rights. The army, like organized religion, maintained a needed psychological weapon by depriving its fighting men of their curls. Like prisoners of war and concentration camp victims, new recruits into Uncle Sam's service were shorn and made to feel as dehumanized as possible, as the first step in the psychological process of building a different social hierarchy. Hair is far too personal a statement to be allowed to assert its power in a supposedly homogeneous group.

We love our hair and hate the thought that someone or something can take it away from us. Whether or not we purposely use its length to make a personal statement—of a political or fashionable nature—we consider it an integral part of who we are. No other part of our body so reaffirms the fact that we are indeed living and growing and changing. When our fingernails grow, we tend to clip them, cut them away as the dead and useless afterthoughts they are, discarding the notion that with each trim, life is passing us by. Our hair is different. When we cut it, we are reaffirming life; we know it will grow again. No matter how bad a hairstyle may look, how much the stylist may bungle a cut—we have the natural buoyance of a new chance at life, of starting over. We reassure ourselves of our hopes with the message, "It will grow out." With each subsequent hairstyle we have another chance to affirm that we are alive and well, growing and changing.

Few people look better without hair. Few balding men go gently into that good night. Pregnancy, illness, diet, stress, and medication can cause thinning or temporary loss of some hair, but most women don't panic until they suspect they are losing a substantial amount of their mane.

The thought of hair loss during cancer treatment is a horrifying one. In fact, many patients report that the mere thought of the loss is much worse than the actual loss itself. Many things in life are worse in the anticipatory stage than in the reality, and for a lot of people, loss of hair is one of those things. For others, hair loss is the ultimate insult. It is a tangible reminder that they have cancer; that they are different; that life is something they have little control over.

If the patient is a breast cancer patient who has just had a mastectomy, the hair loss may be interpreted as yet another assault on her femininity; another intimate part of herself being taken away. "I think I could have dealt with the cancer on my own, private terms," says one patient, "but when I found out about my hair, I went nuts. It's one thing to face your own mortality, but it's another to consider yourself a freak, especially when you're at your lowest."

If the patient has been able to hide her illness from the public, loss of hair announces to the world that something has gone wrong. "Cancer is a very private battle," explains one woman, "especially when it's internal, not like breast cancer where everyone can see your breasts. I had stomach cancer. I felt like it was no one's business but mine and my family's. That was all well and good until my hair started to fall out. You get real defensive when you're trying to be private about your grief and then someone says, "You're wearing a wig, Edna?"

Drugs, Toxins, and Their Effect on Hair

Hair is made out of *keratin*, the same protein that makes up the fingernails. Instead of coming out of the body in sheets, like the nails, it's pushed out from the hair shafts in coils—each coil is a strand of hair. There are actually two types of hair: short vellus on the body, and darker, longer, terminal hair on the scalp. During puberty, the vellus is replaced by terminal hair in the pubic and axillary regions.

The hair on your head is attached by a hair bulb, or root, that is buried in a layer of skin called the *dermal papilla*. Small blood vessels carry hair building blocks to the papilla, where they are changed into keratin, which is a combination of amino acids. The keratin fibers are actually springlike chains of molecules that are bonded together by various other materials including hydrogen, cystine, and sulfur. These chemicals create the actual properties of each shaft of hair, be it curly, wavy, or straight.

There are approximately 100,000 to 130,000 hairs on a head at any given time. There is a natural amount of hair loss in the aging process; between birthdays 20 and 80, an adult can expect to naturally lose about one-fourth of her hair. For this reason, it's very common for women over the age of 65 to gravitate toward wigs or hairpieces to fill in their thinning locks.

In its healthy state, the hair grows according to its own life cycle—each cycle lasts between two and five years. Then the hair goes into a resting stage before it resumes growing. Each shaft of hair has its own cycle, growing at a slightly different rate. Growth also varies according to sex and age. It would take about six or seven years of nontrimmed hair growth for a woman to have waves she could sit on; it would take a middle-aged gentleman a much longer period of time to achieve the same effect.

Hair grows at a different rate on different parts of the body, as well. Even among people of the same age and sex there can be a great variety in rate of growth, although scalp hair seems to grow faster in women than in men. In both sexes, however, the growth rate is highest between ages 50 and 70.

When a patient is receiving chemotherapy, she gets a measured dose of a drug. The point of the treatment is to kill the cancer cells. At present, there are no drugs that just kill cancer cells; chemotherapy affects all cells at once. In general, the cells that divide the most rapidly are affected the most, and cancer cells tend to divide more rapidly than any normal cells in the body. The cells that line the mucous membranes (like mouth, genitalia, rectum, and the gastrointestinal tract) reproduce the fastest and are, therefore, the most affected by chemotherapy; growing hair roots are the second most susceptible. The side effects of chemotherapy are directly related to the type of drug, the amount of the drug given, and the metabolic rate and location of the exposed cells. Although each body reacts differently, there are some rather standard expectations of each drug.

In order for the drug to do its thing to the cancer cells, it must be circulated throughout the body via the bloodstream. As the blood vessels carry the drugs to the hair follicles, the chemicals are so strong that they kill off the productive hair-growing cells and turn off the hair follicle so that it retreats to its resting position. This causes the hair to fall out from the root, but leaves the follicle safe and intact, ready to grow new hair when treatment ceases. Because the drugs are timed to enter the bloodstream when cancer cells may be dividing or growing, the treatment is designed to interfere with "normal" cell proliferation. As long as this process is going on, no new hair can grow.

Loss of hair is called *alopecia* (aloe-PEEsha). Alopecia is usually temporary, but people with a disease called alopecia areata, which is not related to cancer, are unable to grow new hair. Cancer patients who lose hair as a result of chemotherapy treatment usually grow new hair. Patients who have received radiation to the head may not grow new hair or may grow hair of a different texture.

Within two to six weeks of the first chemical treatment, hair begins to fall out. Because each body reacts differently, and because different doses of drugs are given to different patients, the amount of hair that falls out varies on a per-patient basis. Hair regrowth uniformly begins three to five weeks after treatment ends.

Depending on the type of drug and the strength of the dose, hair loss can range from mild thinning to *total* loss of body hair. I mean *everything*. Some patients lose eyebrows and eyelashes as well as pubic hair. Others lose only the hair on their heads. Some have only thinning of the scalp hair. Others lose patches of hair; some of the hair remains, steadfastly holding its ground. Other patients lose all their hair except the wisps around the front hairline.

Before Chemotherapy

One of the most upsetting sentences that patients of both sexes will hear from their doctor after their initial diagnosis is the one that informs them that they may lose their hair. In fact, hair loss has become so tied in with cancer treatment that very commonly the first question a patient asks the doctor after discovering she has cancer is, "Will I lose my hair?"

"As soon as the doctor said it, I knew. In my mind they were the same thing. I couldn't have told you then which one I thought was worse—finding out I had cancer or knowing I would lose my hair," says one patient.

"I kept telling myself to be brave," says another, "but then when he [the doctor] said I would lose my hair, I just came apart."

While you may have very little time between initial suspicion of cancer and surgery, there is often a good bit of time before the chemotherapy treatment begins. (Not all patients have surgery; some begin chemo almost immediately.) Because of the toxic nature of the drugs, and the lowered resistance caused by chemo, doctors want their patients to be fully recovered and healed from their surgery before they undergo chemotherapy. As a result, you may have two to four weeks to stew while you worry about chemo and hair loss. This is unfortunate, because many people fantasize themselves into a dither. Don't be cruel to yourself! You deserve better.

To prepare you for the actual loss, there are several things you can do before you begin chemo. First of all, consider that you have two separate problems to deal with: (1) the outer realities of hair loss—you will need a wig; (2) the inner realities of hair loss—you need to adjust to the loss of your hair so that you suffer the least possible psychological trauma.

Never be embarrassed about your thoughts regarding your hair; never feel the need to keep your grief over the upcoming loss to yourself. "I knew I should be lucky I was alive; that being alive was the important thing," says one woman. "But underneath all that, I couldn't help but be upset about my hair. I didn't want to tell anyone because I thought they would judge me harshly and just tell me to shut up or stop being a baby or to think about the important thing, that I was alive. Something so small as losing my hair seemed minor compared to the fact that, without treatment, I would die, so I felt real stupid even admitting that I cared."

"I felt guilty every time I thought about my hair," said another woman. "I knew in my mind that it shouldn't matter, that it didn't matter. But in my heart, it mattered. And I was ashamed of myself."

If you think you need some professional counseling, seek it. Don't be afraid or ashamed to admit that you're having trouble dealing with the loss of your hair. Proper grieving for your hair *before* it leaves will help you better face the loss at the right time.

While you're allowing yourself the freedom to freak out, give yourself some balance by remembering that most things are worse in the anticipation stage. While you cannot make your fears go away, take some support from the fact that over 65 percent of the women I talked to reported that their hair loss was not nearly as bad as they thought it would be.

When you're ready, have a beauty session with yourself in the privacy of your own bathroom. Make up your face to your party best, and then use a towel or shower cap to secure your hair back away from your face (see photo). Or slick back all your hair with a mousse or gel— just plaster it down so that it becomes invisible against your scalp. Study your face carefully, looking at your good features and then at

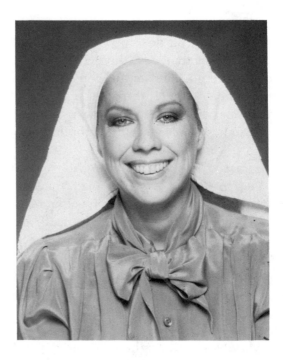

the less good. Learn your face and its structure, without the surrounding hair. Then remove your makeup and repeat the process. This will be less kind. Study the map of your face and accept what you really look like. This visual and emotional acceptance will help you face the day when you look in the mirror and see yourself without hair or makeup. This is the real, the unadorned you. Whether you are a natural beauty or not (and few of us are natural beauties!), coming to terms with the basics will bring you a peace of mind that helps you to cope with the upcoming difficult times.

You may want to repeat these beauty-and-the-beast sessions as often as once a day. They are not meant to depress you. If you find the session to be overwhelming, discontinue it and consider counseling or professional help.

As you come to terms with your face, you may want to start thinking about a wig. You may not experience enough hair loss to need a wig. On the other hand, if you have $50 to spare, you may want to invest in what I call a "beginner's wig." The wig should always be sought before chemo begins.

Before your hair loss, even while you are recovering from surgery, there are some preparatory steps you can take that will make eventual hair loss easier for you later on:

- Get out the yellow pages and look up WIG. Don't fret if there is no listing. Try HAIR REPLACEMENT. Even if there is only one listing, the resource may be perfect for you. After all, you only need one wig. Call and ask how many styles they have to choose from; how long it takes to get new styles; if they have catalogs you can look at, and so forth. Are you happy with the wig selection in your hometown, or do you want to go to a larger nearby city for a better choice? Many women get depressed when they think they will have to make do with a prosthetic device (that's income tax talk for wig) they don't like. Because the loss of your hair is such a psychological issue, you may feel even more damaged if you don't like the selection in your hometown. If a trip to a bigger city is warranted, make plans immediately after you are strong enough, possibly before you begin chemotherapy. Don't allow yourself to panic or get carried away. Some women feel compelled to get to the nearest big city to shop for a wig when, in fact, the selection at home is quite adequate. If you find yourself feeling obsessive about your pre-chemo preparations, consider it a sign of stress and find someone to talk to.

- If you are planning on buying your wig through a mail-order firm, write for the brochures immediately, as it will take a week or so before the catalogs arrive. Make sure you can get a refund if you are not satisfied.

- Once you've bought the beginner's wig, begin to wear it immediately. This will help you and your family adjust to

your new look. Remember, the wig will feel and fit differently once your hair is gone. Wearing the wig before
chemo is an exercise to make you feel more comfortable,
to help you get used to the wig and how you look in it.

- Put together a chemo beauty kit to take with you to the
  hospital or treatment center; make sure there is a wig
  brush or hair pick in the kit.

- Find a favorite *recent* photograph of your natural hair in a
  style that you like and be able to show it to your wig
  consultant. If possible, place a copy of the snapshot in
  your Baseline Beauty Profile. If no such picture exists,
  have a picture taken as soon as possible—an instant picture is fine.

- If your hair is colored, have a consultation with your
  colorist and your doctor. Your doctor may have definite
  opinions on chemically colored hair. If your doctor
  doesn't want you to color your hair again between diagnosis and hair loss, you may want to begin to wear a wig
  to cover color changes in outgrowing hair, before your
  hair begins to fall out.

Fallout

While few women question the necessity of losing their hair, most are
not prepared for the big moment when it happens. Because the fallout
rate is different for each person, most doctors say very little about this
subject. You can ask questions, but no one can answer them with
certainty. Many doctors suggest that their patients have their hair cut
very short before they begin chemo. This helps prepare you for a
change and makes the loss less traumatic, but it can also backfire.

"I had my hair cut like a little boy's," explains one patient, "and I
was totally calm. It looked real cute, it was summer, everything was

fine. I waited and I waited. Nothing. Then, just the back fell out. If I had left my hair long, the top hair would have covered it and I would have looked totally normal. It was like a bad joke."

"I was planning on getting a haircut, but just hadn't gotten around to it. I thought, gee, I've got several weeks 'til it's supposed to go. Three days later, my hair was coming out in hanks. I knew it would fall out, but what a shock!"

For reasons no doctors can yet fully explain, many patients complain of pain when their hair falls out. It's thought that whatever the chemotherapy does to the follicle to cause the release of the hair is also responsible for the pain. The pain is not severe and lasts for a week or two, usually the week the hair actually falls out and the first week thereafter. Some patients have shooting pains, others complain of hot and cold flashes along their scalp. Because the scalp has been protected by hair during most of the patient's lifetime, it is indeed sensitive.

If your head is sore, wear a knit cap that will feel like a soft cuddle. The pressure of the cap helps ease the discomfort.

The Emperor's New Hair

Denial is an important part of our complex psychological state of self-protection. Many women deal with hair loss by denying it. While a few deny that they will have a loss and therefore don't prepare for it, the much more common approach is to live through the loss and deny that it is real.

"I saw pictures of myself bald and burst into tears," says one survivor. "I knew I was bald, I know, but I'd never taken it in emotionally. It was like the emperor's new clothes. I could see hair. Or my image of myself with hair was so strong that when I saw myself without hair, I wasn't really seeing myself."

Although it is healthier to come to grips with your hair loss, it is not necessary. It's much more important to come to grips with your illness. It's better to deny that you have a hair loss and cope with the realities of cancer as you fight back than to deny that you are sick at all.

Acceptable Losses

There are people who deal with their hair loss exceptionally well. In fact, they find the best approach is an aggressive one. Losing their lives is not an acceptable alternative; losing their hair is an acceptable compromise.

I met a cancer patient who lost her hair twice. The first time, she lived through a very traumatic three days during which every hair on her body—except her eyelashes and eyebrows—fell out. "It was the most devastating experience of my life," she recalls now. "I knew it would fall out; I had accepted that. I wasn't feeling sorry for myself. But when it happened, I couldn't believe it. Huge hunks of hair were everywhere. I felt like I was watching my life go out of me right before my very eyes."

Three years later, she had a recurrence that called for more chemotherapy. "It's very hard to lose your hair a second time," she remembers. "You think you were such a good sport the first time, you can't believe you will go through it again. The more I thought about it, the angrier I got. I realized I had lived through not having any hair just fine. What was so terrible was watching it fall out by the handful. The more I thought about it, and I thought about it all the time, the more I wanted some control over my life. I went to my husband's barber and said, "Take it off." He gave me a crew cut and I felt fabulous. When the short hairs fell out, I had no attachment to them. I had won the battle. It was my personal triumph against cancer."

This is not a technique for everyone. First of all, not everyone will lose her hair, so the method may be uncalled for. But for those patients who have a strong possibility of losing most or all of their hair—for those who have already faced the fact that they will have no hair for a portion of their lives, who feel it's better to take control of a situation than to be a victim—getting there first can add a psychological victory that few cancer patients have experienced. It is being the master of your own fate; it is taking control over an area in which you thought you had no control.

If you decide to do this, remember these things:

- Do not have your head shaved to the skin. The possibility of being nicked is too great. Patients who are undergoing chemotherapy will have a lowered white blood cell count and are therefore more open to infection. A nicked scalp, besides not being very attractive, can create serious problems and may actually delay the date on which you start your chemo treatment.

- A barber gives a better—and cheaper—crew cut than a beautician. Practice makes perfect. Just how many crew cuts do you think Vidal Sassoon did in his time? Discuss your decision with several professionals and see how they feel about it. Your regular hairstylist may be terrified to clip you, or delighted. Since this is an intimate act, you may want to share it with someone who knows you and your hair, rather than with a barber you've never seen before. Check it all out first.

- Because this is an unusual practice and a gutsy step, if you discuss with the barber or beautician your reason for taking this step, he may not charge you for the service. Cancer patients are always surprised to find how supportive their hairdressers are at this time of need. Of course, you should expect to pay—especially if you are being clipped by a stranger. Price out the service carefully. I paid $50 for my shave-in-a-haircut in Beverly Hills, while the neighborhood barber told me he would have charged me $10.

- Do not go to a beauty school for this service. The evenness and the finesse of the cut may not matter, but you cannot risk injury to your scalp. Don't take chances with beginners. Likewise, never volunteer to be the first clip your own stylist has done. Barbers have much more experience, but ask them also—a youngish barber may not have performed his quota of crew cuts in this blow-dry era.

- Don't forget to take your wig with you when you sign up for a crew cut. You may want to leave the salon with the same amount of hair you came with. On the other hand, short hair has never been more popular and you may feel perfectly comfortable showing the world your cut. This is up to you.

- Don't hide the crew cut from your family or yourself. You may not want to go to the grocery store or the mall looking like a Marine, but you must deal with your hair loss as a private, family matter.

- Remember that healthy hair grows very quickly. If you get a crew cut before you begin chemo, your hair will grow out before it falls out. Hair grows approximately half an inch a month.

The crew cut is just one stage in the hair loss procedure. When the drugs take effect, your crew will fall out and you will be bald. Accepting yourself with a crew is the first step toward accepting yourself bald. Do a lot of mental homework before and after the crew cut. The crew cut is supposed to make you feel triumphant. If you are unable to get up the courage to take control, do not berate yourself. It takes an awful lot of guts to assault your precious hair. But if you are strong enough to walk into a salon and whack off your locks, there's no question that you are strong enough to be a survivor. You're more than halfway there.

The Crew Cut

Many things are worse imagined than experienced. If you are considering a crew cut, read this section so that you can understand the process. A crew cut will be performed in two stages. (1) The bulk of your hair will be eliminated with an electric razor. This will take less than five minutes and does not hurt. (2) The stylist will change blades and will shave and shape the remaining hair to an even length. This will take ten to twenty minutes and does not hurt, although you will be aware of the vibrations of the razor.

If you want a tail left at the nape or a flat top in the front, advise your stylist *before* the big trim.

Stylists experienced in this kind of cut will usually sit and talk it all over with you before they begin. They'll give you a chance to chicken out, as well.

Keep in mind that if crew cuts are the rage in fashion, as they are in some punk circles now, you may end up with a very insensitive barber. There are currently barbers-cum-stylists whose specialty is shaving, painting, and sculpting very short hair. They consider it an art form. If you need to be treated a little more delicately, find a hairstylist who understands your situation.

Types of Hair Loss

Hair loss due to chemotherapy is quite mysterious: no one can predict with total accuracy who will lose what and when. The type of the drug (not the drug combinations) and the dosage are the factors that most affect hair loss. The higher the dosage, the more complete the hair loss.

Hair loss due to radiotherapy is confined to the area that has been irradiated. It may be a permanent loss; hair may return but not in all its former glory.

Hair loss due to chemotherapy may be full or partial; this is usually a temporary loss. Almost all chemotherapy patients regain their hair.

Often chemotherapy and radiotherapy are given to the same patient, but usually not simultaneously.

Women who are having both radiation and chemotherapy may have radiotherapy first. Many secretly worry that the power of the x-rays will damage their body so that once their hair falls out during chemo, it will not grow back. This is one of those myths based on a half-truth. Most people know, from watching sci-fi movies or antiwar documentaries, that radiation causes hair to fall out. They wrongly assume that radiotherapy is comparable to nuclear fallout, and so they panic. Rest assured, radiotherapy is not anywhere near as potent as the radioactivity in nuclear warfare. Although it is true that if you have radiation to your head, your hair may not grow back, only a small percentage of cancer patients have radiotherapy on their heads. Radiotherapy for breast or ovarian cancer, or for many other types of cancer, will not cause permanent scalp damage.

Hair loss due to radiation will always be specific to the area that is irradiated. Hair loss due to chemotherapy will be more general and more unpredictable. Hair will simply shed of its own accord. When you brush your hair, wash your hair, or shake your head, you will notice significant loss. Hair will come out by the hunk; hair will be on your pillow when you wake up; hair will fall into your food while you are cooking and eating. When you go for a wig consultation, the stylist will touch your head and more hair will fall out. You will have the sensation that if you reached into your scalp you could easily yank every single hair out by the handful.

"My hair was very long at the time, it was my pride and joy," says one woman. "It began to fall out from the back, around the hairline at the nape of my neck. It never did all fall out. But each time more hair fell to the floor, I felt that a piece of me had died."

"I knew my hair would begin to fall out any time," says another, "but until that time I didn't want to look unattractive. So when my roots began to show, I did my hair color just like always. Well, when it came time to rinse away the foam, boy did I get a big surprise! Every single hair on my head rinsed away as well. I was totally, I mean totally, bald!"

"I wish all my hair had fallen out," complained one woman, "and that I hadn't made such a big deal about the whole thing. I was left with these funny little sections here and there that were rather long-ish."

Hair loss is nonspecific. One half of your head does not go bald while the other half stays fine.

Hair loss falls into four patterns:

1. Loss of 25 percent or less of the scalp hair, causing hair to appear thin, but not necessitating a wig

2. Loss of 50 percent or more of the scalp hair, leaving clumps of hair here and there

3. Total scalp baldness

4. Loss of all body hair

Preventing Hair Loss

As chemotherapy becomes more commonly used, doctors and nurses have begun to question chemically induced alopecia. Many have conducted experiments designed to help patients save their hair—or enough hair to make the efforts seem worthwhile.

There has been some experimental work with an enzyme called Q-10 that has been given orally to patients on Adriamycin with excellent results, including some cosmetic advantages. Minoxidil, which is being used topically in a 2 to 3% cream formula by balding men to inhibit male pattern baldness, has not been found effective for cancer patients.

Doctors have also made attempts to save hair by using scalp caps. The basic thinking is that if the bloodflow to the scalp can be reduced, less chemical toxin will reach the hair bulb and fewer hairs will fall out. The first doctors to attempt this procedure used tourniquets, or bandages that were so tightly wrapped that they did indeed cut off part of the circulation. They were also fearfully painful.

In the late 1970s, various teams of doctors and nurses working separately all over the world began to experiment with hypothermia treatments—applying cold to the scalp with the intent to constrict the blood vessels in the scalp, which would allow less blood to get to the hair roots. They used ice at first, but it was messy when it melted and difficult to administer. Since the results showed promise, ice was replaced by gels or cold packs that didn't melt and could be fitted into caps.

Because Adriamycin has traditionally caused the most complete hair loss among its users, most hypothermia experiments have been done on patients whose chemotherapy included this drug. In a study done at the Royal Marsden Hospital in London, nurses found excellent results with patients whose dosage did not exceed 50 milligrams of Adriamycin with each injection.

Scalp caps were created from polyethylene cooling packs that were joined together with waterproof tape (it took seven packs to create the average cap) and then molded to head shape on a wig stand. The caps were stored at −4°F until needed. Patients began their thirty-minute scalp-cooling treatment fifteen minutes prior to their chemotherapy. The best results were found when:

1. The patient's hair was wetted prior to treatment.

2. Ears were wrapped in gauze and cotton muffs to prevent frostbite.

3. The entire head was then bandaged with a wet crepe bandage.

4. The cooling cap was applied while the patient lay back against several pillows. Although the cap weighed about 5 pounds, the pillows gave head, neck, and shoulders support to make the waiting period more comfortable.

Of the thirty-one patients tested at Marsden, twenty-eight tolerated the treatment without side effects or serious complaints. One felt faint and discontinued the cold packs; two other patients were too tired to continue the treatment (as a result of their illness, not the treatment). Some of the twenty-eight successful subjects complained that the cap felt heavy for the first ten minutes; nineteen complained of light-headedness after the pack was removed but felt fine a few minutes later; two patients had shivering attacks that were corrected with extra blankets. The majority of the patients liked the adventure of the experiment and the thought that they would be able to prevent hair loss; all said they enjoyed having the nurse spend the time with them to talk privately and answer questions.

Of the twenty-eight patients who stayed with the program, twelve had no hair loss. Eleven of those twelve lost pubic hair and other body hair, but not the hair on their heads. Ten other patients in the group had minor hair loss, but not enough to need wigs. Thus twenty-two of twenty-eight patients had "socially acceptable" hair loss. The remaining six patients had severe hair loss.

Although hypothermia work such as this is still considered experimental, it is being done in many of the major hospitals all over the world. If such an experiment interests you, talk to your oncologist or your oncological nurse about it, *before* you begin your chemo treatments. WARNING: **Many doctors are opposed to this treatment or any program that constricts blood vessels and inhibits chemical flow. They *want* the chemo to spread to every fraction of the body, to ensure that it can do its job.**

In general, if the cancer is blood-borne or *metastatic*, you do not want to limit the flow of chemicals or chemo in any way. If your tumor was very localized, however, and your doctors are relatively certain there is no more cancer, hair-saving techniques may be discussed as a possibility. Since there is always the risk of occult metastasis—or cancer that is too small to be detected—most doctors feel that hair-saving techniques are not worth it.

Opponents of hypothermal treatments feel very concerned that their patients are getting hung up on a cosmetic question when their lives are at stake. Chemotherapy has yielded excellent results with many patients; it is prescribed to do lifesaving work. Why inhibit its lifesaving possibilities just to keep your hair, which will grow back after treatment anyway?

As for other possible hair-saving measures, doctors are having success with infusion devices that attach to the patient's body (by means of a shoulder or belt holster) and distribute a slow, steady amount of drugs over a longer period of time. This lessens the dosage and provides two benefits to the patient: nausea and vomiting are reduced, as is hair loss. Not every patient qualifies for an infusion device, but experiments with them have been promising. Ask your doctor about the procedure if you are interested in more information.

Now What?

Assuming you receive traditional chemotherapy on an outpatient basis, you will report to the hospital for your treatment approximately every three to six weeks for several hours or days of treatment.

At the hospital, you will be surrounded by patients who wear wigs, scarves, and turbans or sport the "King of Siam" look (this is naturally more popular with men). Some hospitals offer beauty services right on the premises, for inpatients and outpatients. You may want to stop by the beauty shop each month for tips.

If your hair loss is more or less total, you will find that you go through a period of adjustment during which you come to accept yourself as a person without hair. For the most part, patients fall into one of two categories: those who adjust rather quickly to their hair loss and discover that their hair wasn't nearly as important to them as they thought it would be, who feel that their real business is to get on with their treatment and to get well; and those who fall apart over their hair loss because they are not yet able to deal with the far greater issues, with the fact that they have cancer and are seriously ill.

There is nothing anyone can say or do that will help prepare a patient for hair loss. Most patients find the time during which the hair is actually falling out to be the most difficult. Once it is gone, or has stopped shedding, they rally and come to grips with their situation. Obviously, some do better than others. Those few patients who have had their hair cut off voluntarily have done much better psychologically than those who have not—but so few people have practiced this technique that it's hard to make a definitive statement.

"Once my hair stopped falling out," says one patient, "I felt my life turn. At first the hair loss symbolized that I had cancer and was a victim. Once I was bald, instead of being depressed, I got new energy. The hair loss began to symbolize my treatment—that help was available, that I was getting better."

Another patient remembers, "I thought it [hair loss] was going to be some big terrible deal. It wasn't. I wore a scarf a lot and I don't think people even knew. Or if they knew, they acted like they didn't notice. No one ever said, 'Why do you wear a scarf all the time?' People don't care half as much as you think they will. You don't feel nearly as bad as you think you will."

"I always thought it was real interesting to go to the doctor's office and wait for my appointment. I'd look around at all the other patients, and you could tell who was coping and who wasn't just from what they did about their hair. There was one woman all done up very fashionably with a turban and nice makeup on and nothing was going to get her down. She had great spirit, which I admired. Then there were people with scarves tied around them like their grandmother had worn when she'd just gotten off the boat. I thought they were kind of sad. I saw a lot of nice wigs. Very few women had the courage to go without anything, although I did see a beautiful young bald woman wearing a star sticker on her scalp in a very jaunty manner. It made a fashion statement and a bravery statement that I'll always admire. She gave everyone in the office the courage to laugh a little."

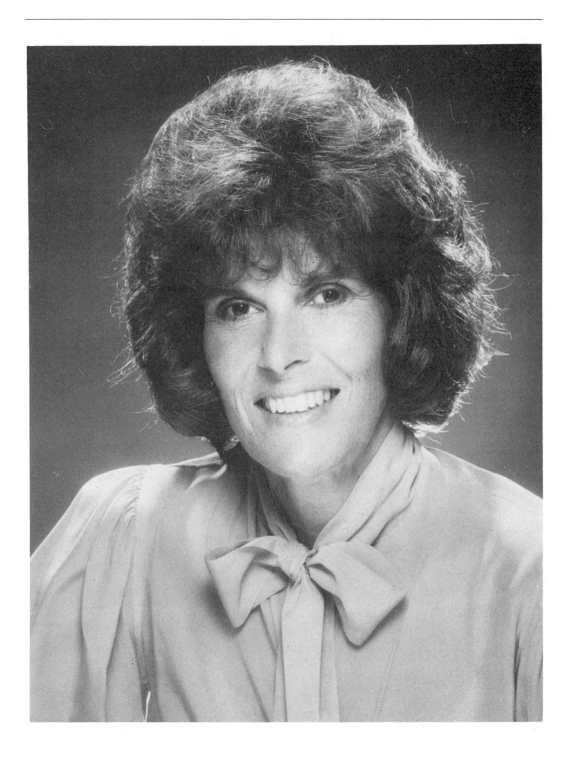

Chapter Three

~-

WIGS AND WITHOUT

To Wig or Not To Wig

The wig is an ancient article of apparel, worn for beauty and status as well as for health reasons since early times. Egyptians wore wigs to keep the midday sun from giving them sunstroke; in Greece both men and women wore them. Wigs became popular for theatrical use in Roman times, and shortly thereafter were established in royal courts (Elizabeth I wore one) and courts of law (English barristers still wear wigs).

Movie stars have always worn wigs, on and off camera. And wigs went into pop fashion in the 1960s when Rudi Gernreich and André Courreges independently showed clothes on models who were synthetically coiffed with glossy black, pink, or green hair.

Although any woman who came of age in the 1960s and early 1970s remembers having a fall, a hairpiece, or a wig or two, these artificial enhancements did not stay in vogue. Today, 90 percent of the white women who buy wigs do so for medical purposes. (Statistics show that black women buy more wigs for fashion purposes.)

Womankind has a long-standing tradition of having hair on the head. Society becomes very nervous when forced into daily commerce with people who do not have hair. Even totally bald men, like Yul Brynner and Telly Savalas, are considered oddities—and that's in a world that knows and claims to accept bald men. There is only one socially accepted bald woman—Persis Khambatta—who rose to fame because she willingly chose to have her head shaved for the movie *Star Trek*. Khambatta may have been the most beautiful bald woman in history, but she did not start a trend. Women all over the world did not rush out to get a Persis 'do, as they had for Irene Castle, Dorothy Hamill, or Farah Fawcett. Let's face it, people just don't like the idea of bald women.

As a result, the cancer patient finds herself under pressure to look "normal"—to wear a wig, or to cover her head in such a way as not to offend the viewing public. It takes a very strong woman to face the world bald.

"I told her not to wear the wig," says one husband of a 52-year-old woman. "She's got a beautiful face, she always has. Here she has cancer and she's being real brave and going through all this treatment like a trooper and she still looks great. If she wants to wear the wig, that's her business. I tried to get her to go without it, but she doesn't want to. If you ask me, she's being foolish about it. When you're as pretty as she is, hair doesn't matter."

"I never, never, never would have gone without my wig. My husband had left me for a 23-year-old girl with lots of hair and a cute little tight body about six months before I found out I had cancer. You think about that for a while. I never had good hair to begin with, and to suddenly lose what I had was just another reminder that I had a special problem."

"People's reactions to me definitely depended on whether I had on my wig or not. When I wore the wig, everyone in my family could cope. They were supportive and understanding. When I took off the wig, it was chaos. Everyone was so upset they fell apart. There was a lot of anger there, too. They were mad at me for getting cancer and doing this to them. I think the people around you want you to hide your problems as much as you can. We end up wearing wigs to protect the feelings of those who love us. The wig is for them, not for us."

Wig Tricks

- The right wig style for you is the one that makes the best of your feature flaws and helps create an illusion.

- If your face is round, do not add to the roundness by picking a wig with a bubblelike hairstyle. Long, straight hair usually makes the face appear longer. Since this style does not look very natural in a wig, opt for a short style that gives height without adding width.

- If your face is narrow at the temples and wider at the jaw, pick a wig with more hair on the top—perhaps fluff or bangs. Feathered layers of hair will widen the appearance of your face and give it the perfect balance we all seek.

- If your face is narrow at the jaw and wide at the temples, or if you have a prominent forehead, pick a wig that frames your face at the ears and nape without adding a lot to the top half of your face.

- If your neck is long, or you are overly thin, you will probably look better with hair at the nape of your neck. Short, short hair is not for everyone.

- Few people look bad in a medium-length hairstyle of soft fluff. If you are at a loss for the right style, begin with the safety of this category.

- Hairstyles convey social messages. Pick a style that represents what you have to say about yourself and that is appropriate for your age. Although it's a total myth that the older you get the shorter you should wear your hair, a 65-year-old grandmother might look a little foolish in a Tina Turner wig.

- You can use mousse or gel on a wig to give it all the fashion pizzazz you want.

- You can wear your wig to a beauty parlor and get a cut, just as if it were real hair. Don't pretend it *is* real hair, however.

- Your wig color must be coordinated with your skin tone if you don't want to look foolish. If you have olive skin, forget about your fantasy of being a platinum blonde. It's just never going to work. If you have white, white skin and think blue-black hair will make you look like Snow

White, you're right—it's a cartoon image, all right. Black wigs are hard to wear even for people with naturally black hair. They should never be worn by women with very pale skin.

- You hair must also be coordinated with your clothes. Don't pick a wig that is so radical a change for you that none of your clothes look right.

Wigging Up

"I love my wig," grins one patient, as she fondly touches her auburn-tinged locks. "It looks far better than I ever anticipated. It's actually better than my own hair. I may use wigs even after my hair comes back. I have a new freedom I never expected. It's faster, it's easier, and I think I look better more often. Now I'm not at the mercy of some hairdresser, either."

"I hate my wig," confides one woman with a very sharp, bitter edge to her voice. "You'd think that at 55 I wouldn't be so vain, but you're never too old to appreciate your best feature. Mine was my hair. It was very full and thick, and I kept it a beautiful red-gold color thanks to Clairol. I never wore much makeup or kept up with fashion or did any fancy treatments to myself. I just always looked nice and simple and had good hair. You can't get that color, or that fullness or that texture, or the confidence from a wig. A wig is a mean thing—it lies there reminding you of what you once were. Even when my hair grew back, the doctor told me not ever to use that kind of hair color again. My real hair was brown and gray and ugly."

"Cancer took away my breast, but more importantly, it took away my sense of myself. It wasn't the mastectomy that did me in; it was the loss of my hair and the knowledge that it could never go back to the way it was. One look in the mirror reminded me that I was a different person. I want the old one back, with or without a breast."

The need for a wig is a painful one, but it can be a positive experience. Because society so very much wants women to have hair on their heads, most patients feel much more secure once they have found a complimentary wig.

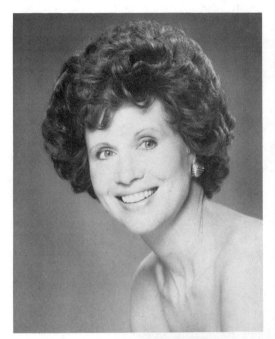
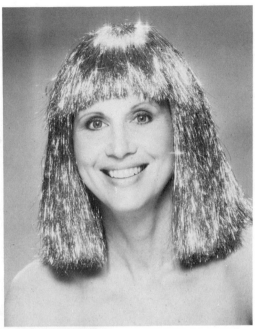
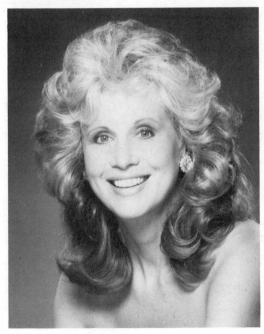

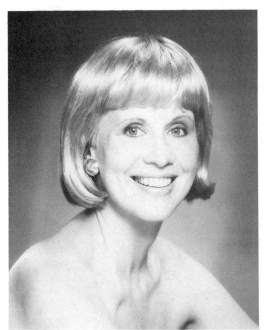
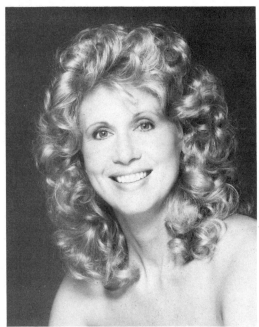
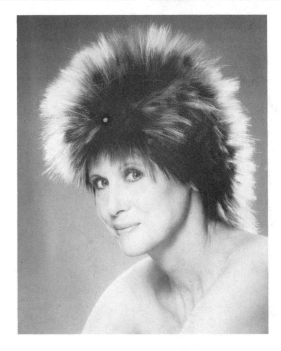

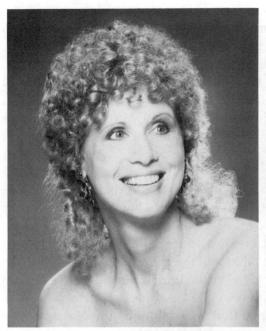

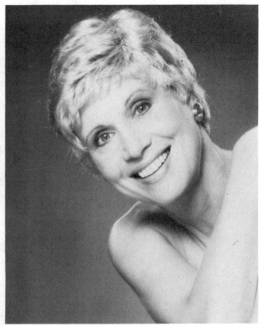

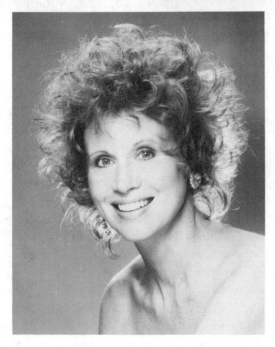

It is virtually impossible for anyone, especially a woman, to say, "Oh, well, I'm going to lose my hair, but it will grow back again" and take a lot of comfort. The loss is an intensely private one, but it is a true loss that everyone experiences. Because it is such a devastatingly difficult emotional issue, many women do not deal with the realities of wigs beforehand. Busy with the sudden change in their lives, they go about their business, reassuring themselves that when the time comes they will get a wig. Few women pause before their hair loss to digest the most important, least avoidable fact about a wig: *A wig is not your hair.*

Many patients expect the wig to look, feel, and react just like their hair. If it doesn't, they chide themselves for not having bought a more expensive model. They think that it is possible for fake hair to look exactly like real hair. In most cases, it is not. Many, many people get good—and inexpensive—wigs that fool the public and make the wearers feel they look their best. On television and in the movies, a wig can look exactly like hair, but it will never be the same as a person's hair—this is a fact of life. Accept it, so that you can enjoy the blessings of a wig. Don't ruin your wig for yourself by demanding of it things it cannot do. Don't tell yourself that you will look exactly the same. You can come extraordinarily close to what you looked like before, depending on hairstyle and type of hair, but there will be slight differences. Enjoy them; don't bemoan them!

These days, the making of wigs is a science and the wigs are quite remarkable. They represent better living through chemistry. For the most part, you can get a full and well-colored synthetic-hair wig for $30 to $50. If you're willing to spend $1000 to $1500, you can get a wig so fine that few will know it isn't homegrown. Although an inexpensive or poorly worn wig can be the cause of anxiety, wigs are basically miracles of crafting that can bring a great joy.

"People come in here with scarves around their heads, feeling defeated," says Bob Akre, a Hollywood, California, hair-replacement specialist. "They walk out wearing a wig and a smile. You can see how much better they feel automatically."

Full wigs are either handmade or machine-made; of synthetic hair or of real human hair. Synthetics are usually machine-made; human hair is usually used in handmade wigs. Hand-tied hair moves in many directions; machine-sewn hair does not. There's a relatively new category of wig, hand-crafted especially for chemo patients; it is made of synthetic hair and retails for about $100. This is a little more expensive than a ready-to-wear wig, but because it's hand-tied, it has greater versatility.

The cost of a wig depends entirely on the two variables. Human hair costs more than synthetic hair, and handmade wigs are more expensive than machine-made ones.

The fashion wig business for white women faded in the mid-1970s. No longer does each American woman over the age of 15 have a wig stand, or two or three, on her bureau. A few young, hip women of the mid-1980s have brightly colored or punk-style wigs for fashion fun, but the days of wearing a wig because it looked better than your own hair are over. Today, wigs are being worn more than they were five, or even three, years ago—and these are fun, fashion wigs that reflect a mood and are considered an accessory to clothes. Women over the age of 35 who would like to try some of the new-wave looks but are afraid they will look ridiculous are now turning to wigs as they did when they were in their early twenties. Wigs aren't strangers to them and they are gladly spending $30 to $50 for a piece of fun. What are they buying? Green, blue, or purple hair, of course.

The Custom-Made Wig

Custom-made wigs are the most expensive and the best wigs a person can buy. The best selections of wig makers are in the large cities and fashion centers of the world. In the United States, they're New York, Los Angeles, Chicago, and Dallas. On the international front, don't forget London and Paris. However, these are not, by any means, the only cities that have artisans who create custom wigs. Although you may want to take a trip to a city that offers the best selection, remember that a custom wig is like a couture dress. You will require at least three fittings before the creation is completed; the wig maker may even make a plaster cast of your head.

On the first meeting, the wig maker will measure your head and take samples of your real hair. At this time you will discuss styles, hopes, dreams, fantasies, and fears. Although a good hand-tied wig can be combed and arranged in any number of styles, you should specify the way you normally wear your hair and what styles you are most adept at. If you have pictures of hairstyles that interest you, or of yourself with your hair in the style you are planning to wear most often, bring them along. The more information you give, the more the wig maker can help you. Remember, with a fine custom-made wig, you will be able to arrange the hair in several styles, as you would your own hair. The main difference will be that the wig doesn't grow. The measurements to be taken include head circumference, forehead to nape, ear to ear over forehead, ear to ear over the top, temple to temple around the back, nape of the neck. If any of these measurements are not taken, leave. And don't come back.

On your second visit, you will try on the unfinished wig cap to ensure that it fits properly. This part gets tricky, because if you still have your hair, you may not get precisely the same fit as you would if you didn't have any hair. Of course, you can space these visits far enough apart so that you have hair for visit number one and don't for visit number two. In terms of fit, this is the ideal situation.

On the third and final visit, the wig is styled while on your head. It may need to be cut a bit, or some small adjustment made. You will be given a few lessons in the care and feeding of your wig, and all your questions will be answered. A well-fitted custom wig should not slip, but you may want to ask about toupee tape if you are worried about it. A custom wig will grab the contours of your scalp and not just sit on top of your head.

Expect to pay $400 to $500 for a custom-made synthetic wig, $1000 to $1500 for a real-hair wig. Do not wear the wig swimming, in the shower, or to a tanning parlor (cancer patients should not go to tanning parlors anyway). A good wig is a fine piece of equipment. Treat it with respect if you expect it to look its best.

Think seriously before you decide on a custom wig; go for a consultation or have some discussions with beauty experts. Few people really need a custom wig when their hair loss is a temporary one.

The Ready-to-Wear Wig

It wasn't long ago that every department store you went to had a wig section where women happily tried on the latest style, for color, cut, or plain old fun. Now that the fashion wig business has dropped off, few department stores carry ready-to-wear wigs. If you walk into your local Saks Fifth Avenue, you will be sorely disappointed to discover that they don't know what you are talking about. Although a few department stores still carry wigs, the best place to find a ready-to-wear wig is a wig store or a private hairdresser who specializes in hair replacement. Mail-order catalogs provide a wider selection than you might find in any wig store. Although you should not buy your first wig through a catalog, mail order can be a happy solution if you find you are successful with a certain brand of wig and want to branch out to another hairstyle or length.

The average wash-and-wear wig costs $30 to $50. It is made in the orient, which is why the price is so reasonable. The U.S.-made version of the very same wig would cost at least $200. There are about half a dozen big firms that distribute ready-to-wear wigs in the United States—among them, General Wig Company (which includes the Adolfo line), Wigs of France (Allen-Arthur), Eva Gabor, and René of Paris. The Eva Gabor wigs are available all over the country and are particularly popular with cancer patients; the Allen-Arthur wigs are equally popular, but are known by several different brand names, Allen-Arthur being just one of the labels that Wigs of France makes. (It also makes a wig specifically for cancer patients, called the Great American Option.) René of Paris sells wholesale and retail and also does private label work. It not only supplies wigs to all American film and television studios but also works with hospitals and burn clinics across the United States. The René of Paris line is sold through wig stores, as are the private lines. General Wig Company is a division of Revlon. It makes wigs for salons, wig shops, and department stores; it produces the Adolfo line of wigs and works directly with some cancer patients. All of these companies make hairpieces as well as full wigs; they do a small amount of business in fun wigs—orange or blue hair, mylar wigs, and the like.

People often buy wigs through mail-order catalogs or from self-service racks in discount stores. One of the best ways to go wig shopping without a catalog is to buy the *Star*, which has numerous ads for wigs—with pictures of many of the styles and a chart for color selection. The prices are incredibly low—just above wholesale. You can get a wig through one of these ads for $20—and many of them are from

Eva Gabor! There are also Eva Gabor wig boutiques, in May Company stores in California. Department stores that would never consider returning to the hair-replacement wig business are now stocking some fun wigs in their first-floor accessories departments, near the hats and the scarves. This is a direct result of the punk fashion look and cannot be expected to last. Wig availability is somewhat related to fashion, but every community has some selection. If you are interested in a wider range than what you find in your hometown, write to the wig companies listed in the back of this book for catalogs or information.

All wig distributors offer the latest in fashion hairstyles. René of Paris stocks up to eighty shades in one hairstyle; many of those shades are blended colorations—say, three shades of gray in one wig for a very natural look, or blonde tones that are lighter around the face and darker at the roots. René personally claims that if you send him a lock of your real hair, he will match it for you exactly, a boast that he says no other company can make.

In a wig shop, expect to pay $50 for an Eva Gabor wig, but watch for sales and closeouts that may drop the price to $25 or less. A René of Paris wig will retail for whatever price the stylist thinks the market can bear. Its average price is also around $50, but René warns that the same wig will have a higher price tag if bought from a fancier salon or a more experienced stylist. The Wigs of France wigs are more expensive—usually in the $100 range—but they come in a cute little fabric box and are packaged much more distinctively than other wigs.

Wig Rip-offs

Cancer patients are extremely vulnerable to rip-off because they long to trust someone who can make their crisis a little bit easier to take. Every now and then, a wig dealer will take measurements and act as if he is preparing a custom wig and then, three weeks later, present the patient with a ready-to-wear wig, but at a custom wig price!

Go only to a wig maker that has been recommended by a hospital, doctor, support organization, or friend.

If a wig costs more than $100, take the time to think about it.

Hairpieces

If the patient retains 25 percent of her hair and just experiences thinning, hairpieces and half-wigs may be the solution. All major wig companies make these.

You can also have a piece made from the hair you have lost. One woman reports that she had been depressed about her appearance as her daughter's wedding day approached, and couldn't stop crying. A friend reminded her that she had been saving the hair as it fell out, and then proceeded to make a series of large curls from the hair. The curls were attached to the thinning places with bobby pins, and the rest of the hair was swept up. The mother of the bride had a very natural looking hairstyle, all made from her own hair. "You gave me back my Anna," said the father of the bride.

If you have a good bit of your hair left, but feel it needs some jazzing up to make you look more like your old self, there are three possibilities: a three-quarter wig, individually inserted hairpieces, or a clip-on hairpiece that is attached to a net that is woven in with your natural hair, to fill out the scalp.

A *three-quarter wig* is much like a fall and attaches to your own hair. When the colors match perfectly, the human eye usually cannot tell where the real hair ends and the fake hair starts. This is very popular for use on camera; few viewers can guess that their favorite movie stars have augmented their locks.

Fringes and switches are popular with movie stars and adapt well to cancer patients. A *fringe* is a front piece of hair—like bangs—that can be attached under a scarf, turban, or hat. A *switch* is a ponytail that can come out from under a hat, turban, or head wrap. Many fashion designers use brilliantly colored switches (yellow, blue, orange) in combination with natural hair in ponytails or braids for their models. You can adapt this idea according to how much hair you have.

A piece called a *clip-on* is very easy to use. It has metal grippers sewn into its web which allow you to attach it to your own hair and not worry about flipping your wig. René of Paris makes these items in all the normal hair colors, but also does some brights. If you're feeling wild, or want to make an outrageous fashion statement, try a burgundy or green clip-on. Your teenage kids will love it. You'll pay $5 to $10 for a clip-on at a beauty supply shop.

If your hair thins, you may want to pull it back to your nape and add an artificial chignon or a twist. You can add fashion accessories and feel quite elegant. Big bows are very stylish now.

Thin-Hair Tricks

For patients who want to make the most of the hair they have left, remember these tricks:

- Don't be afraid to wash your hair. Washing will not make it fall out any more or any faster than it would normally. Clean hair always has a special bounce and fullness.

- Don't treat your hair with chemicals that you think will help it out—no extra conditioners or gels or foams. These tend to build up and cause breakage or damage. Some may contain alcohol, which will dry your hair and make it break off more easily.

- Use a wide-toothed comb, not a brush, and always be gentle when you comb.

- When possible, allow your hair to dry naturally or under lights. Don't use a blow dryer; if you must use a blow dryer, do not overdry.

- Don't use electric rollers.

- When drying your hair, fluff it up from the roots. Shake your head some, or lean your head upside down every now and then for added fullness.

- If your doctor says it's all right, try a nonperoxide hair color or henna treatment. These tend to bulk up the hair a bit. Also, lighter hair does not contrast against the scalp as much as dark hair does.

- Use small inserts or hairpieces. There are many, many types available. Don't be shy.

The Beginner's Wig

If you have made up your mind to get a custom wig, chances are you will already have had your first meeting with the wig maker when you begin your chemotherapy treatment. If your wig is going to be ready when you begin to lose your hair, you will not need—or want—a *beginner's wig* (BW). If your second meeting is to be after your hair loss, then you will need a BW to help you through the first week or so of thinning and/or baldness, until your new wig is finished.

If you adopt a wait-and-see attitude, or have your hair cut away before the chemo begins, you will want a BW—as soon as possible. The beginner's wig is a psychological crutch; it answers that question that you ask yourself in panic each night as you try to fall asleep: "What about my hair?"

The BW should not be a frivolous choice, but even if it doesn't work out for you later, don't ever feel that you wasted your money on this first wig. It will be tax-deductible as a medical prosthesis, but it is even more valuable as a psychological prosthesis, and better for you than all the tranquilizers or antidepressants your doctor can prescribe.

You will be your most anxious when you buy your beginner's wig. This is part of the equation and should be understood and accepted. Buy the BW as soon as you are physically able to do so before your chemotherapy treatment begins. If you have had surgery that keeps you recovering at home, use some of your time in bed to do a little telephone research. Call as many wig resources as possible. (Check the yellow pages under WIGS and HAIR REPLACEMENT; look for the words "experienced with medical hair loss" in any ads.) Call your favorite beautician, ask for information about wigs, selection, services, color range, and price. You may even find that some shop owners or stylists will come to your home to show you a few wigs. Enjoy the process: the more information you have, the better the choice you will make. Even though you may buy other wigs in the future, your BW should not be a foolish choice.

You will be sorely tempted to take someone with you to shop for your BW—or for any future wig. There is one very important rule for this: *Don't.* The last thing you need is someone else's opinion when you are shopping for a wig. Take someone with you when shopping for a breast prosthesis; do not take someone with you when shopping for a wig. Friends and family mean well, but they usually just get in the way. This is between you, your mirror, and the wig specialist. Rely on the wig specialist, who undoubtedly is a licensed cosmetologist (ask), to help you with a wise choice. Don't let the wig be cut for you until you have decided to buy it. Don't let anyone cut a wig on you— so that you can get the right effect—and then pressure you into buying something you feel ambivalent about or don't want.

Choose a wig maker or wig fitter who knows her business. Together you will come up with a solution to your problem. Nothing is more demeaning than having your friends tell you what you should or shouldn't look like at this sensitive, vulnerable time in your life. One of the reasons you are buying a BW is to make mistakes and learn what *not* to do. If the BW doesn't work out, you'll toss it. (Sell it at your next garage sale or put it in the school costume bin; let your children or grandchildren play with it.) You need to choose a wig that you feel good about, not one that someone insists is the real you.

Seek privacy, even for your BW. Do not pop into K mart and call it a wrap. You may do very well there, don't get me wrong, but most wig stylists include their expertise in the price of the wig. They know more than you do. Take them up on it. You are not obligated to buy if a wig remains uncut, so try on many and get a feel for yourself in a wig. There are other reasons for privacy. If your hair is falling out, or gone, you may feel better if you don't have to reveal your condition to everyone around you.

Ideally, your BW will be the same length, color, and style as your own hair. If you can't match your hair shade, go for one lighter rather than darker. If you try on enough wigs, you'll see the difference one shade can make in how you look and feel. (Be sure to have your regular day makeup on when you try on wigs!)

If you happen to have a hairstyle that consists of hair pulled back away from your face, hair trailing down your back, hair placed in a bun or ponytail, or anything without bangs or fluff to it, you will have more trouble finding a natural-looking wig. Consider a change in hairstyle before chemo, and then get a wig that matches your new hairstyle—try for short and fluffy. If you want to go to extremes, it's easy to find wilder-looking wigs, too.

This is not a time to economize. If you tell yourself that a haircut is a waste of money because you will soon lose your hair, you are being too hard on yourself. If you truly can't afford the indulgence, find a beauty college or ask the fanciest salon in town when model night is. Salons always have a model night on which they give free haircuts. You may even want to call a few salons and explain your situation; they just may help out by letting a student practice on you for free. The more you do to help prepare for your hair loss before it occurs, the better you will deal with its reality.

Fashion wigs come in the latest hairstyles—you'll be surprised at how natural they look and how easy they are for you to adapt to. The fluffier a wig, the more natural it will look. Always choose a wig with bangs or soft, short hairs that can be brushed across the forehead. A flat line across the forehead is a dead giveaway that you are wearing a wig.

Once you have bought the BW, begin to wear it.

"I bought my wig with dread," one woman says. "I was so nervous about the whole process that I had to know I had the wig ready and waiting. It was like having the bag packed and in the car when you were ready to give birth. I thought wearing the wig would be terrible. Then one night my own hair looked awful and we were going out and I didn't have the time for electric rollers, so I figured, well, I would just give it a try. So I pulled out this wig that I thought I was going to hate and I wore it, with a little of my own hair brushed out in the front—and it was great! I felt like I looked better than I would have without the wig. Everyone complimented me. I felt funny when someone would say they liked my hair, but then I would just smile and say 'thank you'."

"I have a 5-year-old son," another woman said, "and I had no way of knowing how he would react to my losing my hair from chemo. I didn't want him to look at me one day and think I was a monster or start to cry or do something that would break my heart and make all this worse for me. So when I got my wig, I wore it a lot and left it out a lot. It would be on the bedpost, or on my dresser. I left it in his room one night. He wore it and played with it. He kind of looked like Annie.

My husband tried it on, but of course it didn't fit him. It kind of got to be the family toy and we all had good feelings for it. When my hair started to fall out, I was already wearing the wig a lot of the time anyway, so my little boy didn't notice anything unusual. It took him a couple of days to adjust to my being bald; he would ask me to wear my wig so I would look more like his mommy. But there weren't any traumatic scenes."

Keep a wig diary if you are having trouble adjusting to your BW. Write down the specific problems you are having, as well as your feelings. Later on, in a few months, these notes will help you to choose your next wig. The diary will also help you to adjust to the time when you have no hair and are more dependent on the wig than you are now.

Wigs and Styles

When you think about it carefully, you realize that the reason a person looks so shocking without hair is that the hair fills out the face and changes the shape of the entire head. Models, great beauties, and smart women all over the world have always depended on flattering hairstyles to help them look good. One of the reasons to get a wig in the same style as your hair is that your regular style is probably the best one for your features to begin with. If you've always thought your hair was a disaster, however, this may be a good time to find a better style. The perfect hairstyle plays up your good features and camouflages your bad ones. When you pick a wig, remember this.

Although there is a big difference between styling your own hair and styling a wig (a wig is much, much easier), the people who are happiest with their wigs are the ones who know best how to take care of their own hair. Still, different people have different talents, and certain types of wigs are easier to style than others.

If you are an absolute klutz with your own hair, steer toward an Eva Gabor, Adolfo, or Any D'Avray (Wigs of France) wig. Professionals and people who are good with hair like the René of France wigs the best because they style much more naturally than any other wig—but you need some sense of what you are doing. You don't need to be a

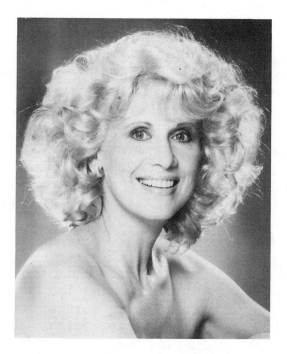

hair genius, but you should be good with your hands. A properly styled René of France wig is indistinguishable from real hair.

Other Wigs

Your BW may be such a success that you find you do not need any other wigs. Many cancer patients buy a second wig not because they are unhappy with the first but simply because they are bored and want to branch out a little bit. A few people buy a second wig that is longer than the first, to simulate growth over the appropriate period of time. Other people feel so confident they begin to experiment with styles or shades that they were not bold enough to try in the beginning.

"I grew up in the Marilyn Monroe years," says one woman, "and secretly I always wanted to be a platinum blond. I never had the nerve to do it, of course. But after I got used to wearing a wig and everyone knew why I was wearing a wig anyway, I decided to live out one more of my fantasies. Having cancer teaches you to take each day at a time, and there didn't seem to be any reason for me not to be a blond bombshell if I wanted to be. It was fun."

A synthetic wig does not have a long lifespan. Depending on how hard you wear your wig, you may find that it needs replacing in four to six months. Wig specialists suggest that each patient have two identical wigs, so that they can be alternated. This makes cleaning easier and provides a little more wear from both wigs. Many people buy a BW and then add a second wig, identical to the BW, later on, when they know the realities of their situation better.

Other women find that they give up wearing their wig very early in their chemo career. They expected to wear a wig full-time when they learned of their hair loss, but for one reason or another have decided to wear other head covers, or go bald. For them a second wig would have been a waste of money.

Patients who can afford to do so often splurge on a third wig—this one is a definite party wig. Either it's in a hairstyle that is not for normal street wear or it's made of an unusual fiber or color. One woman tells me she had bought a pink sweater sewn with plastic angel hair to wear on New Year's Eve. Then she saw a Cleopatra-style wig that was made out of the same pink cellophane fiber that was in the sweater. It cost $50 and she bought it!

"I would have had my hair done for New Year's Eve anyway, and that probably would have cost about $50, so it wasn't a matter of the money. There was just something so silly about this wig that made me do it. When you have cancer you think, 'Well, this might be my last New Year's Eve' or something, so you tend to splurge a little bit more. I thought people would have said I was too old to do something this silly. But I had so much fun doing it that it perked up my spirits. I only wore that wig one other time, and then I gave it to my granddaughter. She still loves it, and I love the memory of how much fun I had in it. Next New Year's Eve I'm wearing my own hair."

If you are looking for an unusual wig but your wig shop only carries the conservative stuff, ask the shop owner. There are trade magazines, catalogs, and beauty shows where many of these items are featured—even if your shop doesn't have something wild in stock, they can get it for you. Because fun wigs are meant to be fun, they usually do not cost more than $50; most are in the $40 to $60 range. You may also want to look in a costume shop, where you can find a fun wig for as little as $10. One woman bought a lime-green Mohawk-style wig for $6 at a party shop and wore it to the hospital for her next treatment. She had fun doing it and gave the other patients and the doctors a welcome laugh.

How to Choose a Wig

Whether you're picking your beginner's wig or a custom job that would be the envy of Dolly Parton, there are a few tips to remember:

- Shop alone. If you feel unsure of yourself or can't make up your mind, take your hairstylist with you. Don't be afraid to walk away and think about it. Let the notion sit with you for hours or days. This *is* an emotional time; you will go through mood swings, and you may feel unsure of yourself. Take your time and make yourself happy. You are the person who counts. Other people's opinions may get in the way. If you're one of those people who can't buy anything alone, do a little research on a wig by yourself before you bring along a partner. Trust your own judgment; always buy the wig that speaks to you. No one else has to wear it.

- Wigs are different from real hair. Think of them that way. They have their pluses and their minuses, just like any other product. Evaluate the way the wig works for you in its job of convincing the public that you have hair. Do not compare it to your own hair, for better or for worse.

- If you've already had some hair loss and are uncomfortable about your looks, seek a wig shop that has private consultation booths. Most do.

- If you are too ill to go out for a wig, ask a wig specialist to come to your home or hospital room. This is not an uncommon request. Some hospitals sell wigs or have their own beauty salons. At M. D. Anderson Hospital and Tumor Institute in Houston, inpatients are given a wig free of charge.

- Get a wig with bangs or front curls that can be softly arranged over the forehead and around the hairline. The first giveaway of a wig is a sharp delineation against the skin. If you have some of your own hair to brush out and style into the wig, this is the best. If you have no hair, pick an appropriate style.

- If deception is your game, choose a wig that is as close to your natural shade as possible, or a little bit lighter. Wig hair colors are specified according to an international number system—the same number is the same color, anyplace in the world. (My color is #30; I have it memorized. Learn your color unless you switch around a lot or use blends.) Blends of these colors may be exclusive to a certain wig maker, but basic shades are all the same.

- Make sure the "scalp" part of the wig is natural. This is especially important for blondes. If you have black skin, get a dark cap to match. A large percentage of fashion wigs are made for black women—you'll have no problem here.

- Black women should know that there are specially made fibers that simulate untreated, natural hair.

- Make sure the wig is not too tight. Many wig caps are adjustable. Others come in three basic sizes, with special large and petite sizes for those who need them. If your wig seller does not have a wide range of sizes but you feel that your head is large enough or small enough to warrant it, ask the shop to order you a specially sized wig.

- If the wig is uncomfortable against your scalp, ask your stylist about a silk or stocking cap. Many hospital supply stores or drugstores sell these for burn victims. You may also want to experiment with the panty part of an old pair of pantyhose: cut off the legs and put the panty on your head, with the elastic framing your face. Then put on the wig. If the panty is way too big, stitch the elastic band or sew the panty into your wig. The new Eva Gabor chemo wig comes with a velvet lining, as do other wigs made especially for cancer patients.

- Wigs of France prides itself on the developments it has made in adhesives. If you are totally bald and worry that your wig may slip, investigate the many types of tapes and "glues." However, worry about wig slippage—or blowing in the wind—is more worry than reality. Most wig wearers do not require tape or adhesive.

Wig Styling

About 70 percent of the people who buy ready-to-wear wigs plop them on their heads and live happily ever after. The rest have their wigs styled. A hairdresser will tell you that you should never consider going in public without first having a wig styled to your face. Nonsense.

Before you get all hung up on styling, be bold. Since styling is usually included in the price of the wig, you may want to shop around. If you don't need the styling, buy your wig from a less expensive source.

If you feel that the wig will be more personalized once it has been styled to your face, choose a wig seller who is also a hairstylist. Most are.

Human-hair wigs must be constantly restyled, set, and treated, just like real hair. It isn't surprising, but it is time-consuming and expensive. Modacrylic wigs have so much bounce cut into the fiber that they style themselves almost automatically.

One of my favorite styling tips comes from the owner of a large wig company. Some wigs, she advises, have to be given a hardy shake, rattle, and roll before you put them on your head. "I can't think of a better way to say this, but shake the crap out of it before you put it on."

It is possible to go to a hairstylist and have him cut a whole new style into your wig. But it will probably cost more than a new wig.

Wig Care

When you buy your wig, ask about its care. You will not wear your wig into the shower, and lather up with your favorite shampoo, but you can take it into the bath with you and give it a light rinse then.

Some specialists will tell you that a wig must be washed with wig shampoo, or brought in to them for special care. An expensive custom wig should indeed get the care its price demands. But a ready-to-wear wig is all wash-and-wear.

"You don't need a wig stand, darling," says Eva Gabor, president of Eva Gabor International "you don't need fancy shampoo. You just wash it and hang it up to dry and shake it, and it's perfect. It's wonderful for travel; it lasts forever. It's very, very easy, darling."

Fill your sink with cool to lukewarm—never hot—water. Add a mild shampoo to the water, not to the fibers of the wig. Then dip the wig in the water, saturating it. If you have used hair spray or gel on your wig, be sure to pay attention to these areas. Add a drop of shampoo to your palms and then wash the wig again. Rinse with clear warm water, not hot. Do not wring the wig. Towel-blot it, and then hang it to dry with a clothespin. If the wig has an open cap, you can use a hanger.

You do not need to use conditioner on your wig, although some wig companies make a chemical conditioner to prolong the life of synthetic hair. This is a very different type of conditioner from the creamy kind you would use on your own hair.

If you have an expensive wig, ask your supplier for care instructions. You may or may not be able to wash it yourself. Use a wig stand to keep the cap in shape. Experiment with rollers; consider having the wig combed out by a professional every now and then, to freshen it up.

Also remember:

- Synthetic wigs will melt (frizzle, actually) if you use electric rollers, curling irons, or electrical devices on them. A hair dryer will not cause meltdown, but it's not advised. Natural air drying is best.

- Wigs usually have more body than your own hair; tease them from the top, not the bottom, and tease lightly. It's not 1964 any more, and besides, heavy teasing will damage the hairs.

- Gels and mousses can be used on synthetic wigs. They're great fun and add a lot of versatility to your styling techniques.

Wig Supplies

When you buy your wig, do not go overboard buying a lot of supplies. If it is a ready-to-wear wig, you need not purchase wig shampoo. You will need a pick and a wig brush—both of these items are readily available in grocery stores and are usually cheaper there than in wig shops. You do not need to buy toupee tape or any product to "glue" the wig to your head.

Wait and see what you really need before buying anything.

Wigless Possibilities

Before your hair goes, you will think that hair loss is a black-and-white matter. You either have hair or you don't have hair; if you don't have hair, you wear a wig. It is not that simple.

There are two main considerations to keep in mind: (1) you don't sleep in a wig, and (2) your wig may be uncomfortable.

As the patient adjusts to the notion of losing her hair, she takes comfort in the fact that there are so many wigs available. If she has already bought her BW, she feels quite secure and on top of the situation. She does not know enough yet or care to dwell on additional harsh realities (or both). She's ready to go.

After the hair loss occurs, the patient loosens up a good bit. Once she comes to accept herself without hair, she realizes that life cannot be lived while hiding under a wig twenty-four hours a day.

I've never yet met a woman who claimed she could have worn her wig all day and well into the night and not thought twice about it. Wigs itch, bite, or cause their presence to be known in a handful of little ways. The average person would like to pull off her wig after a five- to eight-hour stint. People who work in offices or public places manage to get through a workday, but the first thing they do when they get home is kick off their shoes and pull off their wigs.

If you have not yet lost your hair, you will have a hard time understanding that your opinion about hair loss can change after it happens to you. But it will. After a while, you will not be nearly as shy as you think you will be.

If you feel as if you have to hide in a wig, something is wrong. You have not yet come to deal with your illness and should seek professional counseling of some kind. Although having no hair is a deeply personal experience, a woman should feel free to show her naked head to family and close ones. It is nothing to be embarrassed about. Granted, baring baldness is a very intimate act. But this is an important time for you and your loved ones. Don't shut out your family by hiding yourself; don't force yourself into a painful emotional situation when a little love will go a long way.

Going without hair makes a woman feel strangely vulnerable. She waits for reactions, for criticism, even for laughter. She is very aware that people "out there" don't understand or approve. She is terrified that a child will say something cruel.

But there is life without hair, and it is beautiful.

Bald Is Beautiful

In January 1970, designer Rudi Gernreich shocked many when he predicted that in the upcoming decade fashion would dictate a move away from clothes that covered the body. He predicted instead a new interest in the body itself and said that few clothes would be worn, so that the body could be shown off. To make the statement even more explicit, he suggested that men and women alike shave off all their body hair. Bald is beautiful, said Gernreich.

Although he was right about the shift to emphasis on the shape of the body, Gernreich was about fifteen years off about baldness. Only now is it considered a fashion statement for a woman to be without hair. And baldness still is not accepted outside the pages of a high-fashion magazine—say, in the supermarket of your all-American neighborhood.

The time is coming, however, when women will have the option to go bald and make a fashion statement. Alopecia universalis patient Karen Luce says, "I normally just go bald and wear a headband across my forehead. I don't have hair, so why hide it?"

Covered Heads

If you don't want to go bald, try wrapping your head in any of a number of styles, or wear hats. If you are really adventurous, go to the library and study history and costume books to find interesting types of headdresses. Antique shops and foreign handicraft shops may feature unique head wraps as well. Experiment with nonscarf items in your home. Abracadabra, you can be a magician. My most comfortable, easy-to-wrap, and best-looking head wrap was made from a pair of tights. (Plop the waistband around your face, then wrap the legs around your head and tie.) I've made stunning head wraps from T-shirts, sweatshirts, long underwear, collars, and remnants. You have a million resources right in your home; there's no need to run out and spend money on scarves or traditional head wraps that you may never need again.

For those who feel the need to be traditional, here are some options:

The Pookey Cap: One of the easiest things to buy and wear is a little knit cap. Once you have no hair, you notice how cold your head becomes, especially at night. Little Red Riding Hood's grandmother may have slept in a big, frilly bed cap, but today's woman probably sleeps in a

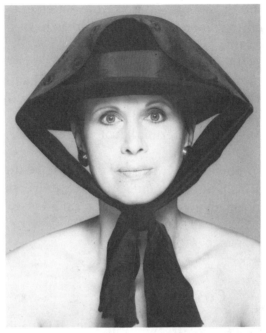

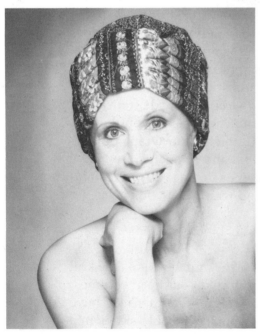

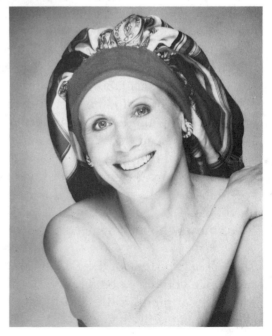

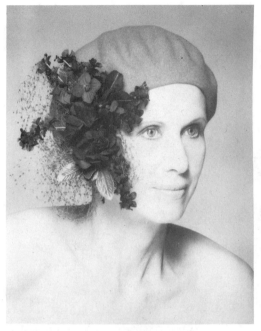
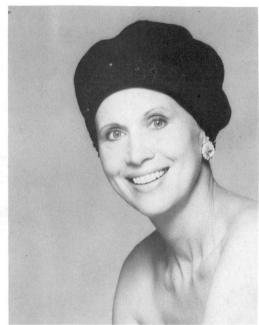
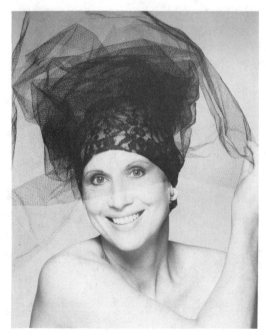
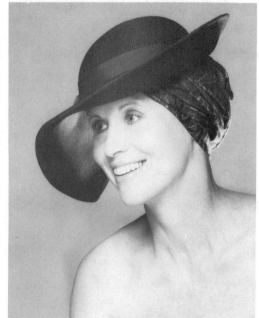

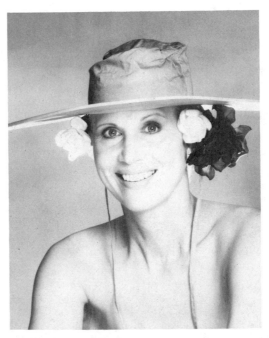

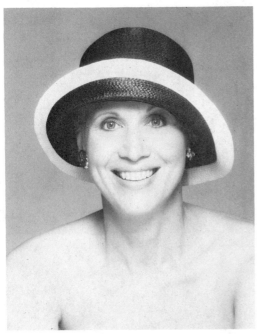

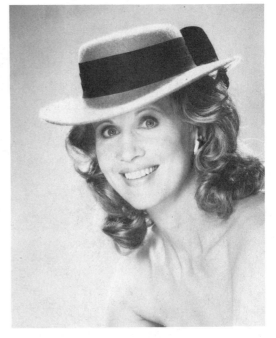

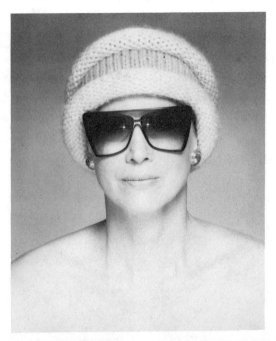

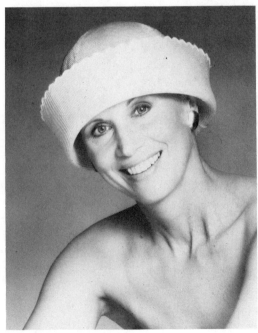

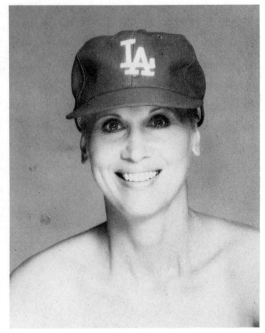

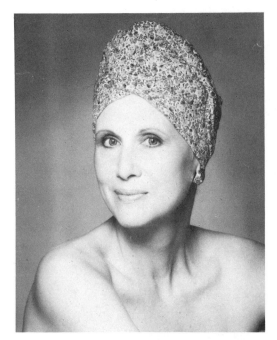
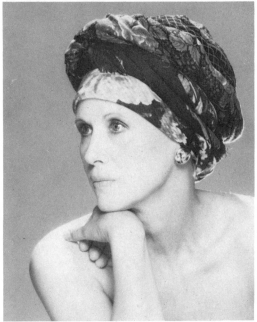
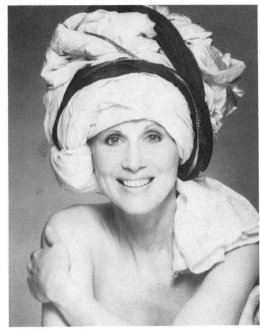

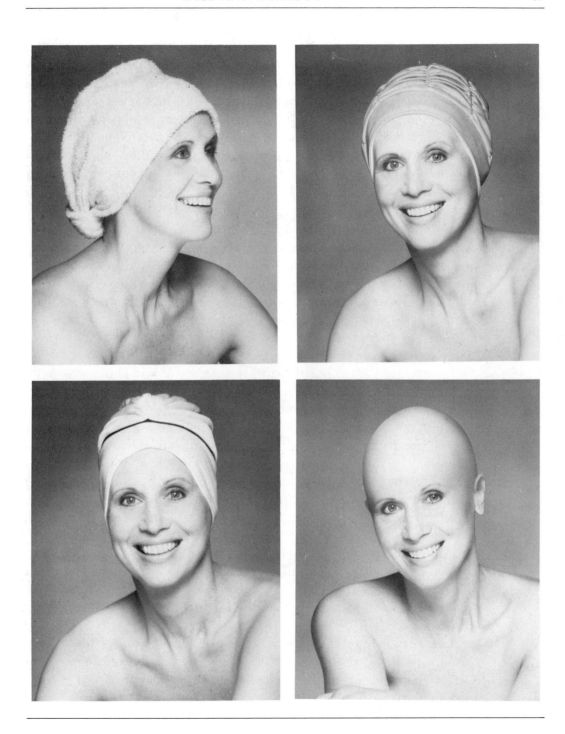

pookey cap. You can buy them year-round, although there is a much larger selection as winter approaches. You can buy the cheapest type—if you're small, try the children's department—at an Army-Navy store, a surplus store, or a dime store for $1 to $4. The navy-blue ones that fishermen wear in TV movies are just fine. You can spend about $10 and get a fashion shade, maybe even in an angora blend. If you are allergic to wool, you will have some difficulty finding a knit cap that doesn't scratch. Buy acrylic. You can also make one out of cotton knit. Or wear a stocking cap underneath.

The Turban: You can buy ready-made turbans, or wrap your own and make turbans to coordinate with your wardrobe. If your idea of a turban is the one you make with a towel when you get out of the shower, think again. Turbans are very, very chic. They are most stylish when they are wrapped several times around the head and have a lot of fabric in them, making them full and high. This does not mean you have to look like Ali Baba.

For about $5 most beauty supply stores and wig shops will sell a ready-made terry cloth turban that comes in a huge variety of colors. You may be tempted to buy these because they are inexpensive, seem like a good idea, and are easy as pie. Yes, they are easy, but if you are used to looking your best, you will not be happy with them—they do not have enough fabric or shape to frame and enhance your face. As a result, they cover your baldness with something worse—blandness. You will look far more pitiful than need be. If these turbans still tempt you, buy one and see how you like it before you invest in one to go with every outfit, or even every nightgown.

You can make your own turbans easily, or have them made for you. The turbans shown on these pages were designed by Nancy Bradstreet, who made them for a friend. All the pattern companies have patterns for turbans.

Get creative in turban making—I've used colored tights (fit the waist around your head and wrap the legs), sweatshirts, old fabrics, and tulle. The two-scarf turban looks best to my eye, it gives you an extra bit of fabric for balance.

The Watteau: French designers have recently shown some very exciting head coverings. They totally cover the head and are largely inspired by the painter Jean-Antoine Watteau. I've nicknamed the cap a "Watteau" and feel it has timeless possibilities for the woman without hair, especially for dress-up.

You may buy a ready-made Watteau, or make your own. Simply cut a circle of fabric—any size from a diameter of 12 to 36 inches—and add a band or some ribbing. Gather the fabric to the band and voilà—glamour. If you make a large-sized Watteau and want a dramatic effect, stuff the inside with tissue paper for a big, full headdress.

The Beret: Who can think of a beret without thinking of the beat generation of the 1950s? Or John Wayne as he immortalized the Green Berets of Vietnam? Perhaps you wore one as a schoolgirl. Maybe you think of Paris. But you've probably never realized that the beret has magnificent possibilities for the hairless. It's inexpensive, soft, and versatile. You can wear it over a head wrap or pull it down to cover your scalp. Several years ago, Sonia Rykiel showed a beret with a veil and proved just how stunning you can look with just a little imagination.

Because this is a real fashion look, you have to have the right wardrobe and panache to carry it off. If you rarely look this jaunty, try adapting the beret to fit your own lifestyle. It's an inexpensive way to be fashionably with-it while you are without it.

The Slink: The slink is a homemade affair that owes a partial debt to Emanuel Ungaro. He sells them for thousands of francs, but you can make one with a yard of fabric. Measure around your head at a line above your brows but covering your ears. Cut the fabric to this length, allowing half an inch for the seam. Close the fabric to form a long bag. Hem the end, or add a border. Stitch four separate straight lines in the hat, gathering fabric as you go. You can gather as loosely or tightly as you want. The finished slink should be about 12 inches in length.

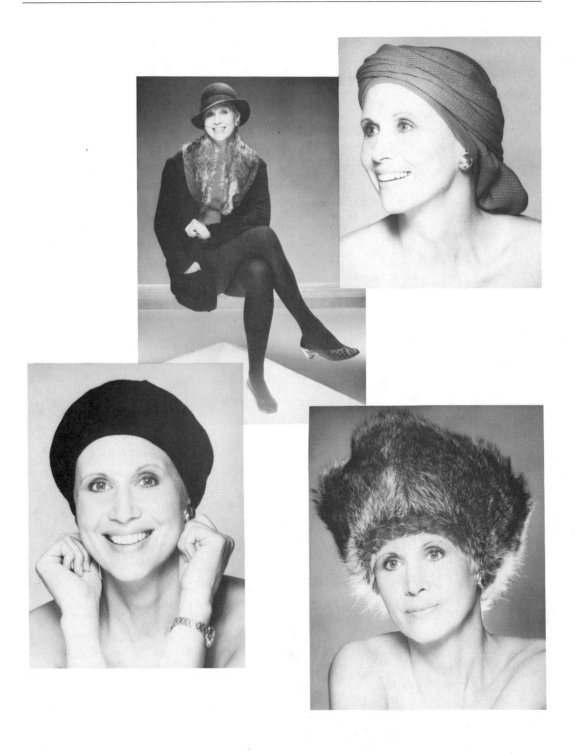

Hat Tricks

Legend has it that the late Coco Chanel always wore a hat in her later years. Always. Mademoiselle was a known eccentric, but the household staff did chatter on about the fact that she even wore her chapeau in the bathtub. As the story goes, when Mademoiselle died, it was discovered that her wig was sewn into her hat!

Today I call that the Coco Chanel hat trick. You can buy a ready-made baseball cap or turban with synthetic hair already attached, or you can imitate Mademoiselle and make your own. (Also realize that a hat properly perched on top of a wig makes the wig look much more real.) Not every hat adapts to the Coco Chanel hat trick, so you'll have to do some experimenting.

Then we have the Katharine Hepburn hat trick. Don't ask me why this hat style reminds me of Kate, but it does. It's a modification of a hat worn in the early 1900s by Edwardian ladies who had to protect themselves from the elements while out in a motorcar. This look works best today for garden parties and teas and can be modified for day wear. It's not great for night.

Don't forget the Yogi Berra hat trick, which comes in two versions—front and back. This sporty look will be preferred by younger women, but is fun for the young at heart, no matter what age. It's also nice when hair begins to grow in. The Yogi Berra hat trick is done with a baseball cap. But, you'll be amazed to know, not all baseball caps are created equal. Do not buy a fashion baseball cap, because it may have a very shallow crown. Also note the proportion of the brim of the cap to the cap part of the cap. The cap should be the bigger part. If the brim is bigger, longer, or more prominent, you have a fashion stylist's idea of a baseball cap and it will not look as good on you. If you're thinking of turning this into the Willy Schumacher hat trick, you can try but you probably won't be satified—jockey caps usually have shallower crowns than baseball caps, and the hairless person needs as much fullness and body in a head covering as possible.

The Popeye the Sailor hat trick is now in vogue. If this hat shape goes out of style, use the photographs in this chapter to have one or more of these hats made: they are ideal for people without hair. The hat does not scratch the scalp (if your scalp is extrasensitive, try the pantyhose trick or a silk cap under the hat) and fits right down to the ears. For summer, choose straw; for fall, there's felt. You can dress it up with a bunch of silk flowers or a glittery pin. I've met several cancer patients who never even wore their wig—they loved this hat so much. Will someone give this designer a can of spinach!

Growing In

About four weeks after your chemo ends, your hair will begin to grow back. It may grow back like a baby's hair—in wisps of cotton candy—or like a man's beard—in stubble. It will not all spring up at once, but will fill in gradually.

The week that the hair actually breaks through the scalp, you may experience discomfort. It is not unusual for the scalp to break out in a bevy of pimples—called *foliculitis,* or inflammation of the hair follicle. Ignore the blemishes, or treat them as you would any other blemish. Do not pick them. Picking these pimples could endanger you life if infection sets in. When the hair breaks through, this is true cause to celebrate. It will be an unusual week for you: emotionally you will be very excited that your body has given the signal that the drugs are out of your system and have done their lifesaving work; physically you may have blemishes and/or discomfort, even shooting pains of hot or cold. A wig that was perfectly comfortable for six months may suddently hurt; your scalp may be very tender.

If your head is sore, you may want to give up your wig for this week and try a head wrap of some sort. Many patients say that they liked something warm, soft, and firm against their scalps—the pressure helped ease the pain. A knit ski cap provides all the necessary elements. It can also be very chic.

The rate at which your hair grows back is related to your age and your general health. If you are in pretty good shape, expect the hair to grow about half an inch a month. During the first six weeks of regrowth, you will experience a very interesting phenomenon: for the first three weeks the hair will seem to grow very fast; for the second three weeks the length of the hair will not appear to change, but the amount of hair on your head will just about double.

Your hair may grow back to look very different from the old hair you knew so well. Some women are shocked to see that their hair has changed color considerably; others are pleased to find that straight hair has turned curly or wavy. Thin hair has been known to come back thick, and vice versa. Many people get what they started out with; but differences are possible.

"I had had perms since I was a child. My mother gave them to me when I was four years old. After I was forty, I suddenly got curly hair—thanks to chemo!"

"My hair has been colored most of my life. When I went away to college it was one color; then, as I got older, I stopped fooling around with it myself, but I always had it frosted in a salon. I got a frosted wig—fine, just fine. When my hair grew in, I thought I would die. I had no idea that it was so dark and ugly and had all that gray in it. After the shock of it, I had to laugh. Of course we get older and our hair gets grayer, but you don't realize it until you start over after chemo. I could be wrong, but I think the chemicals gave me a lot more gray hair than I should have had. But it's a dumb point. I wore the wig, then after about eight months my hair was long enough to get frosted again."

Does She or Doesn't She?

In the mid-1970s there was much controversy over hair dye. Did some colors cause cancer? Should cancer patients not use hair color? As a result of this fuss, some colors were taken off the market and more testing has been done. Most doctors allow their patients to resume hair coloring after regrowth. But don't assume anything. Ask first!

When it comes to chemicals, you must ask your doctor if you are allowed to use hair-color products and what types are permissible. Most doctors are no longer concerned about the use of commercial hair dye.

If your doctor suggests that you limit yourself to a natural product, ask your colorist about henna, a natural root that comes in different colors and in neutral (the neutral is used for added body) and about a brand of colors called Cellophanes. Cellophanes have no dye or peroxide in them—they basically stain the hair. They're great for covering gray and are probably OK with your doctor. Cellophanes cannot lighten your hair, but they do add dimension and body. They wash out slowly over a period of months and never leave "roots." Cellophanes are sold through beauty supply stores or are applied by a professional colorist—you cannot buy them just anywhere. A professional colorist charges about $30. I found it well worth it!

If you are allowed to do anything you want to your hair, consider coloring it after about two months of regrowth, when you will have about one inch of hair. Prior to this time you will merely be dying your scalp, which is unhealthful and unattractive. While the hair is very short, however, you may free yourself from the use of a wig by jazzing up the color with something fun and bright. You may find yourself the hit of the in crowd.

"My hair was crew-cut length and I was wearing a wig," explains one mother of two teenagers. "Then I saw this music video with some punk rock-and-roll start on it whom I had never heard of. Talk about feeling old. First I thought it was a man, then it turned out to be a woman with a crew cut that was bright red. 'That's what you need, Mom,' said one of my girls, we all laughed. But the more I thought about it, the more I realized that hair color would add a touch of fun to my hair. It would look like I had chosen to have short hair; instead of being a victim, I could be a star. I went to a beauty shop where the kids go and got a reddish-burgundy rinse put on my crew cut. I thought I'd die laughing when I saw myself. But you know what? It cheered me up a lot. The kids loved it, and I think a lot of my friends were envious that I had the nerve to do it. We all laughed, but my friends who didn't have cancer kept asking a lot of questions. I could tell they were thinking about doing it too, just to look smart."

"I thought the growing-out time was a good time to experiment," another woman says, "I was wearing a wig anyway. My friends all knew why. I wanted to do something daring for once in my life—to have hair the color of Pam Ewing's on Dallas. That's not such a wild fantasy, is it? So I took a couple of pictures of Victoria Principal to the hairdresser and asked the colorist to make my hair that color. I figured if it was terrible, I would just keep wearing the wig and no one would know the difference. Turns out that I loved it. It was wild and wonderful. It also made the growing-out time a lot more fun."

Perms

If your hair comes back just the way it was and you feel you're going to need a permanent wave again, give yourself—and your hair—a break; don't do it yet. Once new growth begins, wait at least six months before putting any strong chemicals on your hair (this includes hair straighteners). If you can wait a year, do so. Your hair and your body have been through a tremendous workout. Let the fresh, new hair have a good, healthy start before you give it another dose of chemicals.

Virgin Hair

As new hair grows in, you will have the rare opportunity to once more have virgin hair—hair that has not been permed or colored or treated harshly in any way. This is a good time to consider all the hair care mistakes you have made and to reassess just what you want to put your hair through.

Your hair will absorb chemicals thirstily—don't abuse it with color or perms. Expect your old hair color to take differently the first time it's applied to virgin hair.

- Eat well to nourish your hair.

- Don't wash your hair too frequently—twice a week with short, virgin hair should be sufficient.

- Use mild shampoos, and alternate them.

- Condition your hair once it's a few inches long. Don't overcondition.

- Avoid hair dryers unless you must use them.

- Keep your hair covered in the sun; this keeps it from burning.

- Guard against chlorine damage when you swim in a pool.

Private Matters

When the doctor tells a woman she will lose her hair, she immediately thinks of the hair on her head. When she fixates on her impending hair loss, it is to mourn the hair that everyone sees. She rarely even realizes that she may also lose her pubic hair. She rarely understands just how important to her the hair that no one sees can be.

Not everyone loses pubic hair. When it does fall out, however, it's a terrible shock. First of all, many doctors do not specifically say "and that means your pubic hair too" when they explain the possibilities of hair loss, so there is the surprise element. Then there's the fact that the hair comes out in hunks, so that you may go to the bathroom and get an alarming surprise.

Most importantly, few people talk about the emotional value of pubic hair. Our pubic hair was a prize hard won in adolescence—it marked our coming of age as women. We imagine our bodies always with pubic hair, not without it. We feel naked, shy, ugly, embarrassed when we have no pubic hair. For many, it is worse than losing the scalp hair. Having pubic hair reaffirms the fact that we are women; losing pubic hair reduces us to a nakedness we associate with young girls. It's yet another insult that we were not prepared for.

There is no good way to prepare yourself for any hair loss, especially the more private variety. The fact that few people will see you in all your nakedness is not consolation enough. There is one trick I've learned, that may amuse you—but do get your doctor's approval before you try it.

Models who show off bathing suits must eliminate most of their pubic hair lest it straggle out and embarrass them. Indeed, you've probably shaved or used a depilatory for the summer season. The shaving you do, however, is probably minimal compared to what swimsuit models do. Most of them get rid of everything except a small, neat triangle of hair. This entails the removal of about three-quarters of the pubic hair. There are a few reasons why you should emulate a model at this time of your life: (1) Getting used to yourself with less hair will help you with the shock of losing all you hair, (2) it's a very sexy look that you may enjoy, and (3) if emulating a swimsuit model seems foolish, it will make you laugh—and this is a very good time in your life for a few laughs.

Note that your pubic hair will probably grow in again once treatment is stopped.

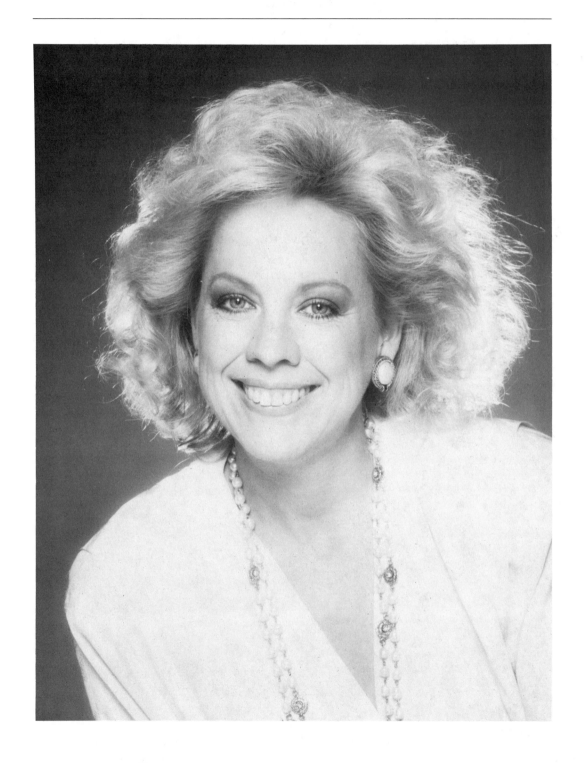

~~~~~~

Chapter Four

SKIN AND MAKEUP

Skin Facts

We've all got it, and got lots of it. Skin is us. The amount of skin on a body obviously depends on just how big the body is, but on an average, a newborn arrives with 2500 square centimeters at birth and as an adult has some 18,000 square centimeters. The average adult male carries 4.8 kilograms of skin, whereas a woman has a mere 3.2 kilograms. And yes, the most important thing you learned in fifth-grade science really is true—skin *is* the largest organ in your body.

Skin is not there just to display blemishes, wrinkles, or a great tan—it has many valuable functions. Skin controls the loss of bodily fluids, prevents penetration of many foreign items, cushions against shock, regulates heat loss, and even sends out sexual and chemical messages to passersby. It is also an important source of sensory information about the environment. Many women consider their skin a barometer of the aging process; for cancer patients the skin is a barometer of the therapeutic process.

The skin is made up of several layers comprising a *dermis* and an *epidermis*, or top layer. The dermis is thicker and is made up mostly of connective tissue. The layers of skin are of particular interest to cancer patients because the patient must become adept at identifying epidermal signals so that the skin does not fissure and open up through the dermal layer. While a hangnail, a scratch or scrape, some peeling skin, or a minor abrasion is not an important wound for the average person, the person who is undergoing chemotherapy is not average. These and other open skin sores (including bug bites and burns) are to be avoided as much as possible. The reason is simple: The patient undergoing chemotherapy has a lower white blood count than the average person. White blood cells function as the body's natural immune system; they attack germs to prevent infection. If you don't have as many white blood cells as you should, your body is open to infection and may not have the wherewithal to recover. Thus a mere cut, bruise, bite, or burn can turn into a life-threatening situation.

"I guess it's just a nervous habit of mine, but I'm a scratcher. I scratch my scalp with my fingernails when I'm reading, or thinking, or talking on the telephone, or even when I'm driving the car. It's not something I ever thought about or realized I did until I ended up in the hospital in an intensive care unit. I don't even know the name of what I ended up with, but sure enough, I got this infection from scratching my scalp. And I could have died because I wasn't thinking. It doesn't matter whether you beat cancer or not if you die of infection. Believe me, it was a real bad scare."

The most important skin tip that you, the cancer patient, can remember is one that mother probably passed on to you when you were 12 years old: *Don't pick.* Mother gave you these words of advice to prevent acne scars; doctors now give you this tip in order to help you save your life. Once you begin chemotherapy, don't take risks. Likewise, before you begin chemo, make sure you are healed. This includes dental work. If you have open sores (even athlete's foot) as you are beginning chemo, show them to your doctor. If you suffer from hemorrhoids, don't be shy, tell your doctor now—they can be a real problem.

Any opening in the body offers a greater possibility of infection and serious crisis. The rules are strict:

- Prevent dry skin from cracking open.
- Never pick blemishes or sores; never bite your lips.

If your white blood count is 1000 or less:

- Don't scratch bug bites.
- Don't clip cuticles.
- Don't use or have abrasive skin treatments (such as an exfoliant or facial) or skin treatments in general; don't use a loofah mitt when you bathe.

The Effects of Treatment

Radiotherapy and chemotherapy often cause changes in the skin of a cancer patient, although each patient reacts differently to her treatment. The most common types of reactions are dry skin, burns (from radiation), rashes, hyperpigmentation (darkening of the skin), phototoxic reactions (reactions to sunlight), and irritations near veins. *Many patients suffer none of these.* They just breeze right through.

The effects of therapy on the skin, however, are the first sign you will probably have that your body is reacting to treatment. Take this to heart and be pleased! The chemicals are making their way through your body and doing their job. Rejoice. The process of getting well has truly begun. Whatever cosmetic problems the drugs may cause you will probably end soon after treatment stops.

If you are receiving radiotherapy, you may develop what doctors call *radiodermatitis*—skin change due to radiotherapy. Skin changes may begin immediately or a number of weeks after treatment has begun. A change may be as minor as a slight drying of the skin, or a scaliness that you would not think twice about if you were not a cancer patient. Some type of dry skin is common for most patients, but this is not necessarily an overwhelming problem. Early detection leads to prevention. Be on the lookout for skin changes, such as dryness, cracks, or tenderness. Mark changes on your beauty profile and report them immediately to your doctor.

Some radiotherapy patients get the opposite of dryness—they experience what is called a "wet" reaction. It's characterized by a weeping of the skin, an oozing that occurs because the top layers of the skin have been burned by the radiation. This is a radiation burn. Do not attempt to treat this condition yourself. If it occurs, tell your radiologist, oncologist, or nurse and get proper care. You may be given a prescription drug or an over-the-counter ointment; you will probably be given a product that is used to treat regular burns, since weeping is a common burn-related condition. A "wet" reaction to radiotherapy is not nearly as common as a dry one and does require special treatment, possibly even temporary discontinuation of therapy. Do not pick at oozing or layered skin. Do not lick it or suck it.

With chemotherapy, the most common skin reaction is dryness, but other conditions affect some patients.

Possible Skin-Related
Side Effects from Anticancer Drugs

DRY SKIN
Adriamycin

Busulfan

Chlorambucil

Methotrexate

HYPERPIGMENTATION
Adriamycin (more frequent in black patients)

Bleomycin

Cyclophosphamide

5-Fluorouracil

Mechlorethamine (topical)

Nitrosoureas (topical)

RADIATION BURNS
(CHEMOTHERAPY-RELATED)
Actinomycin D

Doxorubicin

5-Fluorouracil

Hydroxyurea

RASHES
Actinomycin D

Bleomycin

Mithramycin

TENDERNESS ON PALMS AND SOLES

Bleomycin

Cytosine arabinoside

Methotrexate

Dry Skin

Whether your skin type is oily, dry, or a combination, chemotherapy will probably cause some dry skin. The reaction may be just a little flaking, or dryness to the point of snap, crackle, and pop—resulting in open sores that may have all sorts of fancy medical names, such as xerosis, eczema, eczema craquelé, and asteatotic eczema. These demand serious medical consideration. The skin is an organ with rapidly dividing cells that normally die and flake off. Chemotherapy is especially felt in the skin because chemotherapy is most likely to affect rapidly dividing cells. Many patients have no complaints about their skin during chemo or radiation. Others notice a skin change as the first side effect of treatment.

For average dry skin, the kind that does not open, there are two basic treatments: (1) bathe less frequently and (2) moisturize, moisturize, moisturize.

Bathing less frequently can be your secret (most Americans over-bathe anyway) and will do a lot to help your skin condition. Even if you use a moisturizing machine, you will not be able to protect yourself as much as you can by simply not bathing. Use a washcloth for private cleanliness and call it a day. Definitely do not soak leisurely in the tub. If and when you do shower, make it a quickie. If you can't live without a hot, relaxing bath, or are rewarding yourself with one as a special treat, cover your arms and legs with a protective coating before getting into the water—try Vaseline petroleum jelly or Aquaphor. Use bath oil in the water for added protection. (*Note:* If you are weak, ask for assistance in getting in and out of tubs. The use of bath oils and body lotions can create a slippery condition.) Petroleum jelly will not do too much for getting you clean and will have to be removed with soap (which is drying), but if it will allow you the indulgence of a bath. Also remember that the hotter the water, the more drying it is.

Use a special moisturizing cleansing bar (like Neutrogena or Aveenobar) rather than your plain, old-fashioned soap. These cleansing bars are much less alkaline than soap and will give you a tad more protection. Whatever you do, don't accept or give yourself an alcohol rubdown. Put oil-based products in your bath, but not alcohol-based ones. The most important rule of bathing is to apply creams immediately following your soak to minimize the drying effect of water evaporating from the skin. Use hand lotion after you rinse dishes. Use lotions constantly.

You may want to experiment a bit with lotions and creams to find the right moisturizer for your body. You need not run out and buy a top-of-the-line cosmetic product and smear $75 worth of goo all over yourself each week to properly moisturize your skin. In fact, save the fancy moisturizers for your face and find something cheaper and thicker for the rest of your body. Vaseline will do the trick very nicely, but it's so greasy you'll find that clothes and sheets stick to you. Aquaphor and Eucerin are good, but are extremely greasy. Nivea lotion is liked by more people. Choose a lotion that has 5% lactic acid—LactiCare is a brand of body lotion that a lot of doctors recommend; however, it can irritate. Because creams are thicker than lotions, they may offer better body protection. However, if they are too thick for you, lotion will do the job. Apply as often as possible without being neurotic. Should you develop blemishes, do not assume automatically that the blemishes are from the moisturizer (often they are a coincidental skin reaction), but discontinue creams and call your doctor immediately.

"My hairdresser told me to treat my scalp with a moisturizer because it was flaky and dry," explains one patient, "so that's what I did. I was using a thick cream, every night. It made me feel good to apply the cream because I thought it might also help my hair when it grew back in. Well, a couple of weeks later I got these pimples on my head, like all over. Real embarrassing. Like teenage years all over again, except on my poor bald head. I figured it was from all the grease I was putting on my scalp, so I stopped doing it. The pimples didn't go away and I didn't know what to do about them. Finally I told my doctor. It turned out that lots of people get pimples when their hair is about to grow back and this had had nothing at all to do with the moisturizer."

Dryness on your face can be treated with a cosmetic or dermatologic product created for dry skin. The price of the product has nothing to do with its effectiveness. Just because you have cancer does not mean you need a $50 moisturizer. Buy small sizes of moisturizers to experiment with. Ask your doctor, or your dermatologist, if he recommends a certain product. Many patients find Complex 15, an over-the-counter dermatologic product, to be far superior to anything cosmetic firms offer in pretty jars. Check out traditionally thick moisturizing creams that are considered by the average person to be too heavy for day wear—they may be great for you now. Albolene cream is great for removing makeup.

Rashes and Red Skin

Rashes are referred to as *erythema* by doctors and are common to chemo patients. Skin may also be red without bumps.

"Any lumps or bumps should be reported to your doctor immediately," advises Dr. Arnold W. Klein of Beverly Hills. While rashes are not uncommon side effects of chemotherapy, a rash may also be the indication of an allergic reaction to a certain type of medication. The allergy can be so severe that the patient must discontinue use of that drug and use another in its place. So it is imperative that you tell your doctor of any skin irritations the moment you notice them.

A rash may be restricted to the palms and soles of the feet or to a specific site, or it may be distributed all over the body in a random pattern. With some drugs, the face or chest is the targeted area. Sores inside the mouth are very common also. On the face, you can expect anything from flushing to hives to peeling.

Open eruptions are not common, but sometimes occur. They are more serious than old-fashioned pimples because of the possibilities for infection. By all means *do not scratch or pick* at any rash or sore, whether created by the chemotherapy or by the real world (this includes bug bites!). Mark your Baseline Beauty Profile and report the condition to your doctor.

Hyperpigmentation

Hyperpigmentation is the abnormal deepening of the color of the skin. Although skin color is somewhat affected by the blood and the fat which are part of its composition, the predominant factor in skin color is pigment, or *melanin*. Skin color is both hereditary and environmental. Certain skin tones are common to particular families and ethnic groups; other factors, such as sun (tan), hormones (skin color changes are common in pregnancy), chemotherapy, and radiotherapy, can further affect skin tone. Some skin color changes in cancer patients are restricted to exposed areas of the body (especially true in radiotherapy); other changes may appear as stripes, spots, or bands. Most color changes that occur during cancer treatment fade entirely, or almost entirely (by 80 percent), after treatment. If the color change was caused by a change in the melanin of the skin, it's possible that a dermatologist can bleach that skin back to its original shade, or at least reduce the side effect. If the color change was caused by a chemical reaction, a lightening agent will be of no use. Hyperpigmentation is most common at radiation sites, in the nails (see Chapter Five), at veins where infusion devices have been used, in sun-exposed areas, and in mucous membranes. If you have been pregnant, you may have already experienced a similar reaction called the "mask of pregnancy." Hyperpigmentation is usually not a serious cosmetic problem.

"I was getting 5-FU (5-fluorouracil) and got these really awful brown spots on my face, like age spots but pretty big," complains one patient. "I was really upset about them. I asked my doctor if he could find another drug that would do just as well for my kind of cancer and not give me this kind of side effect. I don't want to sound ridiculously vain at a time like this, but I was very, very upset about those spots. They were all over. I discontinued the medicine."

Hypopigmentation, or the abnormal lightening of the color of the skin, occurs with the use of some drugs. Hypopigmentation of the eyelashes and skin around the eye has been reported in connection with the use of some drugs to treat eye cancer or skin cancer near the eye.

Both hyperpigmentation and hypopigmentation can often be cosmetically corrected with camouflage makeup.

Phototoxicity

Phototoxicity is the fancy term for an exaggerated sunburn response. The drugs that most commonly cause photosensitivity are 5-fluorouracil, methotrexate, vinblastine, and dacarbazine. Be sure to ask your doctor about sun care. Many doctors do not want their patients sun-bathing, playing sports, or even driving in bright sunlight unless they are properly protected. Since sun exposure is directly related to skin cancer anyway, you should use a sun block as part of your regular routine. It's unlikely that your doctor will allow you to use the services of a tanning parlor or tanning device. A block with a sun protection factor (SPF) of 15 will protect you during sports activities outdoors. Reapply frequently.

Temporary Damage versus Permanent Damage

Most skin irritations disappear, almost magically, within three to six weeks after cessation of treatment. Stripes or spots usually fade over six to twelve months. Although some of these pigment changes never disappear, a good number of them become less noticeable with time. If you are not satisfied with your improvement one year after the end of your treatment, discuss your options with a dermatologist. Hyper-pigmentation has been proved to be dose-related. If your drug dosage has caused permanent changes in your skin, but has also kept you alive, give some serious thought to how much you want to complain.

Skin that has changed as a result of the accumulation of melanin may lighten but will be more or less permanent; skin that has changed as a result of the accumulation of certain chemical elements may fade in time, but usually not completely.

In certain cases, radiotherapy causes secondary skin cancer at some point after treatment. Always be aware of any changes in your skin. Check your Baseline Beauty Profile and give yourself a careful once-over every year on your birthday. If you have a personal or family history of skin cancer, check yourself more frequently.

Radiant Irradiated Skin

Radiotherapy offers a rigorous course of treatment. Most patients have treatment every day for a specified period of time. They feel tired, possibly depressed, and are often unable to eat. Weight loss is common. They often do not feel very beautiful and may wonder if they will regain their former good looks. Not to worry. Within weeks after the end of treatment, your appetite and energy will return and you will get your old zippity doo dah back.

Accept the fact that this may not be one of your more gorgeous periods in life, but keep your spirits up with makeup and a strong fighting attitude. Take especially good care of your skin.

Radiation patients with skin reactions should:

- Avoid washing the irradiated area of the skin.

- Avoid use of soap, ointments, or powder near the irradiated area.

- Protect the area from sunlight, usually by covering it. *Do not apply sunscreen without your doctor's permission.*

- Keep the irradiated area dry, but moisturize constantly. Use the simplest products available (Vaseline or Eucerin or Aquaphor).

- Avoid trauma to the skin; tape, bandages, and even rough clothing can be irritating.

Scars: Camouflage and Treatment

A cancer patient may scar for different reasons: (1) from surgery directly related to the cancer; (2) from treatment methods—for example, the use of BCG (now relatively infrequent) or the insertion of an infusion device; or (3) from radiation.

Scars of any type can usually be made more attractive by the injection of collagen—a procedure that must be done by a qualified specialist only after your oncologist has given his permission.

Collagen was recently approved by the Food and Drug Administration (FDA) and is being used by specially trained dermatologists and plastic surgeons for various types of cosmetic work—from filling in acne scars to smoothing out birth defects and plumping up wrinkles. *Collagen* is a natural body material found in cartilage. Currently, bovine collagen is used in injections. Once inserted under the skin, the collagen becomes a fleshlike substance that—much like molding clay—

fills in spaces. Burn scars and surgical scars treated with collagen have shown a 60 to 70 percent cosmetic impovement. Before you get all excited, remember that some people are allergic to collagen—you will be required to have a skin test to see if you can tolerate the treatment. Also, no one knows how long the collagen will stay in place before it begins to dissolve into the body—perhaps a few years, perhaps six months. This can get pretty expensive over the course of thirty years.

Patients who wish to do so or who are not interested in trying collagen may opt to have their scars removed or reduced by a plastic surgeon at a later date. Lung cancer patients have been known to have cosmetic surgery on their scars after they pass the five-year mark.

Scars can also be camouflaged through the use of makeup (see photos). Covermark, Dermablend, and Natural Cover are the three leading brands. Most patients say they prefer Dermablend, but all kinds of makeup are available nationwide at beauty supply stores, some department stores, and frequently through mail order. For excellent coverage that is not as heavy as that of camouflage makeup, try theatrical makeup—this usually has a beeswax base to give it some staying power and may cover your scar to perfection. Blasco and Tuttle are two of the leading brands. You will find the addresses of the companies in the Resource List in the back of the book.

If you have an unattractive scar, splurge on a consultation with the best makeup artist you can get to. You might consider making a trip to New York or Hollywood. For the price of one session (usually $100 to $500), you will learn how to hide your scars and look your best. You do not need to spend $500 to $1000 for a topflight makeup artist, but if you are seriously thinking about it, watch for credits in fashion magazines to find one whose work you admire. Also investigate cosmetological paramedics—cosmeticians specifically trained to work with people who have birth defects, burns, and handicaps. Remember that you can often get free advice from professionals who visit department stores and give demonstrations.

WARNING: **Do not attempt to cover, camouflage, or apply makeup to a scar that is not totally healed. Scabs, crusts, or skin flecks should not exist when you apply any type of makeup whatsoever.**

Camouflage makeups are made differently from regular makeups since they have a serious job to perform. Most are created to color or shade the skin, to resist water and perspiration and lend to the skin an

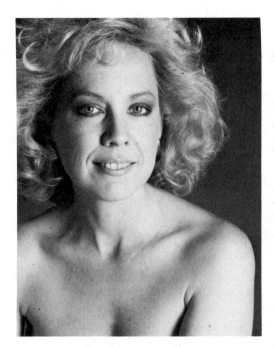 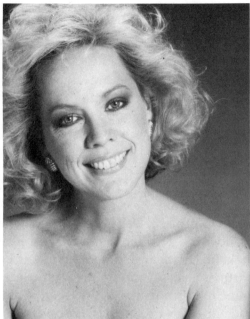

opaque surface that is more perfect than the skin itself. Camouflage makeup isn't meant to blend in with your skin, but to sit on top of it and present a new view of the real you to the public. The bases come in either cream or stick form, and many are used with a special powder that sets the foundation and makes it last longer once on the face. It works best if the entire area rather than a portion of it is covered with a camouflage product—if you have a scar on your neck, don't just cover the scar but work the entire neck area for a smooth finish and unity of color. If the problem is on a larger section of the body—a leg or an arm—limit application to the practical and immediate area.

Skin Cancers

Skin cancer is the most common form of cancer in the United States; over 500,000 cases will be reported this year. It may be a primary diagnosis—your only brush with malignancy—or a secondary one—a side effect of treatment or a recurrence of your internal cancer that has evidenced itself on your skin.

But the good news is very good indeed: over 95 percent of all cancers which are primarily on the skin (excluding malignant melanomas) are completely curable.

The leading cause of skin cancer is overexposure to sunlight, although there are other agents that are known to promote some skin cancers. The most prevalent type of skin cancer is *basal cell carcinoma,* which is a very slow-growing disease. It can take several forms but is easily spotted and can be treated by a doctor before serious damage to life or limb is done. Carefully note changes in skin color or texture and report them to your doctor.

Squamous cell carcinoma is a faster-growing but much less common form of cancer, which attacks the hair follicles and internal skin ducts. The skin usually gives its owner some warning of this type of cancer in a precancerous condition. Check lips, face, neck, and areas of the body most often exposed to the sun—report changes on your Baseline Beauty Profile and to your doctor. Be especially aware of sores that take a long time or refuse to heal. Do not pick!

Malignant Melanoma

The most dangerous type of skin cancer is called *melanoma.* Melanoma does not hurt, grows very silently and swiftly, and kills quickly. It is not a secondary condition.

Malignant melanoma may be related to sunlight and tends to occur more frequently on the normally covered parts of the body which are exposed to the sun during sunbathing. People who live closer to the equator have a higher incidence of melanoma, as do people with light skin, light eyes, and indoor occupations. There is no reason to believe that cancer patients undergoing chemotherapy or radiotherapy have a greater susceptibility to malignant melanoma than any other group of people. Yet, some forms of cancer (such as Hodgkin's disease) are associated with increased risk of melanoma.

The Skin Cancer Foundation offers these tips for spotting a melanoma. Look for:

1. Change in size: a sudden increase in the size of a mole or birthmark should be of concern. Slow change is more common.

2. Change in color: beware of the sudden darkening of brown or black shades in moles or birthmarks, or of the mixing of red, white, and blue shades.

3. Change in surface characteristics: watch for scaliness, flaking, oozing, crusting, ulceration, bleeding, or bulging.

4. Change in consistency: take note of moles or birthmarks that get hard, soft, or lumpy.

5. Change in shape or outline: an irregular border that used to be regular is a danger signal, as is the sudden elevation of a surface that used to be flat.

6. Change in the surrounding skin: spread of pigment from a mole into skin that used to look normal is abnormal. Redness and swelling are other danger signs.

7. Change in sensation: itching, tenderness, pain.

8. Change in pigmentation: Sudden appearance of a new pigmented spot in an area that heretofore has not had such a spot.

If that list seems painfully long to learn and a little bit frightening, try the ABCDs of melanoma:

Asymmetry: if you drew a line down the center of a mole, the sides would not be equal.

Border: the border of a mole or birthmark has changed shape.

Color: the color of a mole or birthmark has changed.

Diameter: the diameter of the questionable mole or birthmark is larger than 6 millimeters.

The ABCDs represent the danger signals of melanoma. Learn them. Remember, almost all skin cancers can be cured if they are discovered early enough. Whatever scars are caused by the removal of malignant skin can be cosmetically corrected at a later date.

Sun Care

One of the best ways to protect yourself from skin cancer—of any kind—is to care for your skin when it is exposed to direct sunlight. Every man, woman, and child should use a sun block of 15 SPF. (Numbers higher than 15 are basically meaningless.) Apply sun block generously and frequently—you tend to sweat it off. Always reapply when you get out of water after a swim. Moisturizers that come with sunscreens in them may not provide the protection you need. If the SPF number is lower than 15, use additional sun block. Two layers of SPF 8 do not equal the protection of SPF 16. Apply SPF 15 over a moisturizer of SPF 8. Then apply your foundation shade.

Radiation patients must stay out of the sun completely.

Makeup

Everyone looks better with makeup. We look better not only to the outside world, but also to our inner self. Unless you have had surgery or treatment on your face and neck, there is no reason why you cannot wear makeup while you are in the hospital and as you battle the forces of evil within.

In the Appendix you will find a makeup chart that can be filled in and torn from this book. If you are hospitalized and run out of makeup, give this form to a friend or family member, who can then buy you precisely the product that you like. Meanwhile, pack yourself a small "chemokit" of your favorite beauty products, which you can stuff in your handbag for visits to and from the hospital. Some days you may feel too ill to touch up your makeup; other days you'll find that a little bit of makeup takes you a long way toward feeling better.

If you feel like makeup, but feel too weak to apply it yourself, ask the nurse or the nurse's aide if she can help you. Some nurses will curtly tell you that they have no time, others will be happy to help out. This varies according to the individual; just don't let your sensitive feelings get hurt if your request is turned down. Figure "nothing ventured, nothing gained," and ask. One of my mottoes in this kind of situation: All they can say is no.

If you are receiving treatment on an outpatient basis, here are a few tips that are guaranteed to make you feel a little bit better:

- *Do* put on makeup before you leave home. Looking better will help you to feel better. If you already have a history of severe illness after treatments, do not use mascara. That way, if you go home and go to bed you won't have to worry about mascara getting into your eyes and causing an infection. If you have been using the mascara with thickening flecks in it, avoid it now.

- *Don't* use fragrance before treatment. You will soon develop a mental link between your fragrance and chemo, and it may actually turn your stomach to smell the fragrance at another time.

- *Do* plan to have some diversion while you are receiving treatment: bring with you a headset and tapes, a book, or a friend you haven't seen in a long time and want to catch up with.

- *Do* freshen up your lipstick immediately after treatment. Use a thick, glossy, possibly flavored listick—this will help keep your lips lubricated, give you a pleasant taste, and make you feel a little more feminine right before things get rocky. The lipstick will probably wear off before the nausea begins; however, if you begin to associate the smell of the lipstick with the nausea, change to an unscented or unflavored lipstick.

Inpatient Makeup

Some people really are too sick to wear makeup in the hospital. If you are one of them, you know it. Otherwise, there is no reason why you can't or shouldn't wear makeup, and every reason why you should. Makeup will help you look and feel better sooner. It should be considered as much a recovery tool as bandages and aspirin. If you desire makeup but feel too weak to apply it, ask a nurse, a nurse's aide, or a volunteer to help you. In the near future, in many hospitals there will be special consultants whose job it is to come around and help you with makeup. As we inch our way toward that enlightened time, we just have to punt and make do.

- There's no need to wear makeup into the operating room, athough some people feel this shows how much spunk they have. In reality, because you will be sleeping a lot after surgery and won't be able to remove your makeup properly, it will eventually clog your pores and do your skin more harm than good.

- Do not treat yourself to a presurgery manicure. Most hospitals will remove your nail polish before surgery, because they like to check on the natural color of your nails as an indication of your health. Get the manicure *after* surgery. Some hospitals even have manicurists who will come to your room.

- Do wear lipstick or gloss into the operating room (and at all times after the surgery), unless you are having oral surgery. This will help keep your lips from drying out and will make you feel a little dressed up for this special occasion.

- If you insist on makeup in the operating room, do not wear mascara. The chance is too great that it will get into your eyes while you sleep in the recovery room. An eye infection is the last thing you need right now, right?

- You will know when you are strong enough for makeup after recovery. This is an individual matter and very often a psychological one. Ask yourself if you are strong enough to reach for your makeup bag...for a lipstick...for a fashion magazine. Interest in these subjects will give you a good sense of your returning beauty awareness.

- While you are recovering, leaf through women's magazines and fashion magazines and tear out ads for new makeup products you'd like to try. A new makeup is a spirit lifter for most women. Consider a new shade or, better yet, a new type of applicator. If you are amused by the new roll-on nail polish, ask someone to bring you one in the hospital. They only cost $3.50—they are a great gift and a great pick-me-up. To make people keep buying products they don't need, cosmetics firms must constantly dream up new gimmicks. Most of them are ingenious and not very expensive. Enjoy. Try something new for the very sake of being daring.

Outpatient Makeup

As soon as you are strong enough, there's no reason why you can't return to your regular makeup. (If you've had face surgery, consult your doctor first.) Just never put makeup on an open wound.

When you begin radiotherapy or chemotherapy, you may find yourself tired (a common side effect from both treatments) and nauseous—not feeling glamorous or wanting to do much about jazzing up your looks. Try to fight the impulse to curl up and hide. Makeup will make you feel a lot better. The ability to wear makeup each day tells you that you are coping. Now is when you need it—so go for it.

"It's hard to feel radiant when you're sick, but if you just keep telling yourself that beauty comes from within, you'll be all right. I went in big for pampering myself to get that psychological edge. I went to a makeup artist, something I had always dreamed of doing; I had a masseuse come to the house—another fantasy. I spent all my savings doing one special thing for myself each month, right after my chemo, so that I felt I was fighting back and winning," says a breast cancer patient.

The most important thing to remember is to keep putting on makeup and doing everything you can to make yourself look as normal and natural as possible. This helps your family and friends, as well as yourself. Looking good is the best revenge.

- If you wear a wig, put on moisturizer and foundation first, and then put on your wig before making up the rest of your face. The proportions of your face will appear different without hair; you will be tempted to put blush in the wrong place if you make up your face without your hair on.

- If you have no hair and do not wear a wig, your makeup should be subtly different. Eyes should be made up a bit more heavily to make them stand out more. Cheeks can be more dramatic, with blush stretching from higher up on the temples, where you once had hair. Be sure to carefully blend your neck, throat, and nape—you can get a much more noticeable line from makeup when you don't have hair at the nape to guide you. Do not put foundation on your scalp unless you are appearing on stage or screen. Blend carefully at the forehead so that you have no color bands.

- Use sunscreen (SPF 15) on your face, hands, and scalp as well as on any other parts of your body that will be exposed to sunlight for more than fifteen minutes a day. Scalp protection is essential.

- Try double moisturing: Use a moisturizer on your skin as always; then mix your foundation with another moisturizer in your palm and apply to the face with fingertips or sponge. This will guarantee extra protection against dryness and a light, sheer makeup that glides smoothly over your face. No matter what your age, this is not a time for heavy, caked-on foundation, which tends to make you look sicker. A moisturizer or foundation that comes with sunscreen already mixed into it may or may not provide adequate protection. Check the label carefully. (See Sun Care, above.) A layer of sunscreen might also act as a moisturizer if it's in emulsion form; however, sunscreen can be drying, so apply it over a base of another moisturizer. You may need sunblock as well as makeup with sunscreen.

- Switch to a cream foundation if you now use liquid. Cream, even when mixed with moisturizer, will give you better coverage. Do not use water-based makeup because it is drying. Some creams in compact form are very easy to apply; use a sponge to keep them light and smooth.

- To help set your makeup and give you a little more color, dust yourself lightly with loose powder; a translucent powder that offers a little shimmer is the best kind because it will help you appear more healthy—it gives the skin a little of that glow that you need right now. You can give your scalp a brief dusting if you don't wear a wig. Be sure to get to your neck—all sides—and under the chin. Use a large makeup brush for this; do not grind the powder into your skin. Don't apply powder around the eye; this may make them look older by accentuating the dry skin in this area.

- If you have circles under your eyes, or brown spots on your skin, camouflage these after applying your moisturizer and before the dusting of powder. For cover-ups use a heavier foundation—preferably in stick form—that matches your own skin tone. Do not go lighter or you will look weird and blotchy. Don't apply undereye camouflage in a half circle; you'll look like a panda or raccoon. Instead, place a dab of cover in the center of the area, and then blend toward the nose. Investigate the various brands of camouflage and theatrical makeup.

- If your skin is flushed from treatment or you are having a photosensitive reaction but are still allowed by your doctor to wear makeup, try one of the creams that enhance and correct off-tone skin. For a reddish complexion, use a green tone. Clinique makes a great one.

- Do not use an eyelash curler while you are having chemotherapy. Whether you lose your eyelashes or not, don't play around with this part of your anatomy now. An eyelash curler creates a trauma your lashes do not need. Not using an eyelash curler will not prevent lashes from coming out, however.

- Do not use mascara with lengthening agents in it—these agents usually consist of flecks that come off as the makeup wears during the day. Flecks can fall into your eye and cause an infection. Bad news. Mascaras are being made in colored formulas—blue or violet, for example—to add a little extra color to your face. If your lashes are fragile or are thinning, just put mascara on the tips. Mascara is drying; removing mascara at night causes trauma to the lashes and can make them fall out faster. Do not have your lashes dyed as an alternative; the dye is much too strong for your lashes now.

- Do not put any eye makeup inside your eye. It is common practice for many to line the eyes with color along the inside rim—this offers more opportunity for infection and is a great big no-no for anyone on chemotherapy.

- If you do not have eyelashes, discuss eye makeup with your doctor. One of the major jobs eyelashes perform for us is to protect the eyes from incoming debris. If you lack this protective shield, your doctor may advise against any eye makeup at all—or he may suggest the simplest of color streaks set back away from the lower lids. If you have no lashes and the doctor allows it, use soft pencil eyeliner along the rim of your eyes to give them better definition and color. Use black, gray, or brown pencil, and then smudge it with a tiny sponge; blur the line and keep it soft. Always do this carefully so that you don't poke yourself in the eye. *Get your doctor's permission first.* Your doctor may suggest that you wear false eyelashes. (See Chapter Five.)

- If you do not have eyebrows, you can draw some in with a little practice. Or you can buy a set for about $15. These must be applied with spirit gum. Pencils are easier. Liz Taylor hasn't changed her style of eyebrows in thirty-five years—so don't worry about penciled brows. And don't worry about having to find the right place on your forehead to draw two lines. When your brows fall out, they will leave behind little dots showing where they once were. This will be your guideline. Using blond or gray pencil, make dots and dashes rather than a firm arch. Practice will help this along.

- Make eyebrows one or two shades lighter than the color of your hair or wig. Do not make them darker than your hair unless you are a platinum or very light blond. The paler your skin and hair, the less defined the eyebrow strokes should be.

- Apply blusher in two layers. The first should be cream. Blend well with a sponge. Then dust over it with a powder blusher. This will do two things: it will help your makeup stay on longer, and it will make your "blush" appear to come from within the skin, as it would for any healthy person.

- If your skin is very lined from weight loss sustained during treatment, do not worry about it. When you are well again, you will regain the weight and your face will fill out, eliminating most of the wrinkles. In the meantime, however, consider one of the creams that temporarily fill in lines and that can be used under your foundation. The results do not last, but may make you feel better. You can use a child's paintbrush (a soft one); fill in your most obvious wrinkles with camouflage, and then top this with foundation. Careful blending is the key to making camouflage effective.

- Don't wash your face with soap. Use a cleansing bar like Dove or Neutrogena or a cream like Albolene. Do not remove makeup with soap and water, but use an oil-based cream or makeup remover. Pat off excess oil with a damp washcloth. Never use astringent while you are receiving chemotheraphy—both are drying.

- Use a humidifier at night. Keep the air moist to help keep your skin moist.

- Never use an abrasive or exfoliating product on your skin. This may open sensitive skin and leave room for infection. Let hair regrowth be your clue that your body is coming back into its own—then use old products that you feel you need. Stay away from anything that will make you peel until your doctor OK's its use.

- A moisturizing mask may be relaxing and temporarily beneficial. Never use an astringent or clay mask to extract dirt—the skin is too dry from chemo for this process. Avoid peel-off masks, because in sloughing dead cells they will remove a layer of skin. This is not the time to be removing anything from your skin.

- If your wig is a new shade for you, remember to buy new makeup. Many women use the chemo period as a chance to try a new hair color with a wig. Skin tone and hair color are closely matched when Mother Nature does the ground-work—make sure that your wig color goes with your skin tone and that you coordinate your makeup colors appropriately. If you have doubts, get a makeup consultation from a pro. If you've had your "colors" done, pick a wig and your makeup shades accordingly. Continue to coordinate with your swatches; remember that while hair color changes with wigs, skin tone does not.

The Two-Minute Face

We all live busy lives, now made even more busy by the demands of doctors' appointments and treatment sessions. It's hard to find the time for makeup; sometimes it's hard to find the energy.

Find it. Reaching for the makeup is one of the most important things you can do to help yourself get better. But you needn't spend twenty minutes getting gorgeous in order to sit on a bench in a treatment center for hours. In fact, if your average makeup procedure takes more than five minutes, you should probably rethink it.

If you're not feeling your best, here's a quickie makeup that can be done in two minutes flat—even if you are flat on your back.

Step One: Apply moisturizer and base. The trick: you have already mixed up what I call Suzy's Blend. Buy one of those inexpensive plastic jars in the drugstore, the kind with the pink plastic screw-on cap. This is the shortish one, about an inch deep and an inch and a half in diameter. Fill the jar about half full with a creamy moisturizer. (I use Complex 15, given to me by my dermatologist.) Then fill about one-fourth the total capacity of the jar with sunscreen (SPF 15, of course). I use Johnson & Johnson. Blend well with finger or plastic appliance. Then slowly add your foundation—in cream form—blending constantly. Test to get the right shade. Once this is mixed, you will have a very light, easy-to-apply makeup that moisturizes, screens, and provides foundation with one application. Use it once a day, and stir before using—it may or may not separate, depending on the ingredients in your products. Apply with fingertips, blend with a sponge. This blend glides on so easily that you can apply it to your face with or without a mirror. (Tip: If you are not using a mirror, blend carefully with the sponge at the nostrils, chin line, and forehead.) Once the blend is made, the time it takes to open the jar, stir, and apply the foundation should not be more than thirty seconds.

Step Two: Blusher. If you haven't got time for a cream and a powder blush, make do with either one. If you are particularly under the weather, the powder blusher will be easier to apply. Find one that comes in a light iridescent shade for some extra shimmer—this makes for a healthy glow.

Step Three: Brighten eyelids with a cream color. If you're too ill to do a full five-minute face, you can still look lovely with only a spot of color to add some depth and zip to your eyes. Buy a cream shadow in a color you enjoy other than plum or navy blue—these will make your eyes look bruised. If you have blue or green eyes, don't use blue or green shadow but try something soft and smoky. Brown eyes can be high-lighted with a warm taupe or even a peachy gold shade. Contrast will brighten up your face and make the eyes look bigger, wider, and brighter. You're trying to add fun and light to your face, but avoid looking like a clown. Dab a circle of color on the lids. Blend if necessary with fingertips. Color should not glare like a stoplight, but should not be blended into oblivion. Keep the circle centered on the lid, not ex-tending past the outer edge of the eye or too close to the nose.

If you have the energy, add a second color by shadowing the crease. This is easily done with a pencil color. Plums, violets, and taupes work nicely for most eye shades.

Step Four: Line eyes with a soft pencil in the color of your choice. You may choose this color to coordinate with your clothes, eyes, or the color of the shadow. The liner should be in a darker color than the shadow but does not need to be black or brown. Some of the eyeliner pencils with the word "kohl" in their name are the best for this. Blend the line, with a sponge tip or cotton swab, for a soft frame to the eyes. You may want to try liquid eyeliner, which is making a comeback. If your hands shake or you are confined to bed, you may have trouble with this. It's not a must-do. Line your eyes using whatever method is easiest for you; do line the upper and lower lids.

Step Five: Apply mascara. One of the gifts I often give friends who have cancer is a Lancôme mascara, shade Marin. It's an electric blue that no one over the age of 25 would ever buy. It's just the thing to perk up your spirits and make you feel a little bit wild. If not now, when? Do not saturate every lash with mascara, but rather lightly brush the wand once across the tips of the lashes—this gives you color and drama without damaging your lashes. Mascara is drying and your lashes are vulnerable now. Go easy.

The Two-Second Blush

If it's just not your day, or you are in the hospital and feeling lousy, you can pick up your looks and your spirits with a mere double flick of the wrists. Use a translucent, pearlized powder blusher (buy a shade that suits your skin color and keep it in your chemo kit) and dust your cheekbones, forehead, and chin. Voilà. Then some lipstick. Smile. You'll feel better tomorrow.

Makeovers

Have you ever dreamed of being a makeover in a magazine? Most of us have. Certainly no one could be more deserving of a few new tips and a sprucing-up than a cancer patient undergoing or recovering from chemotherapy.

I put together a fantasy makeover team and got together with Dr. Herb Rappoport, who lent me a few of his patients. We shot four photographs of each woman: Walk in the Door Before, Old Wig Before, Au Naturel Before and After a session with several of Hollywood's finest makeup and hair experts.

Josef Scigliamo and Maurgerite White from Eva Gabor International supplied wigs and styling services. Sachi of Michaeljohn came with her scissors and rollers to give first haircuts to those who were coming out from under wigs. Marilyn Young rescheduled her celebrity clients in order to do the makeup. We worked with four women: two coming out from under wigs and two in need of new wigs.

Sharon Torres

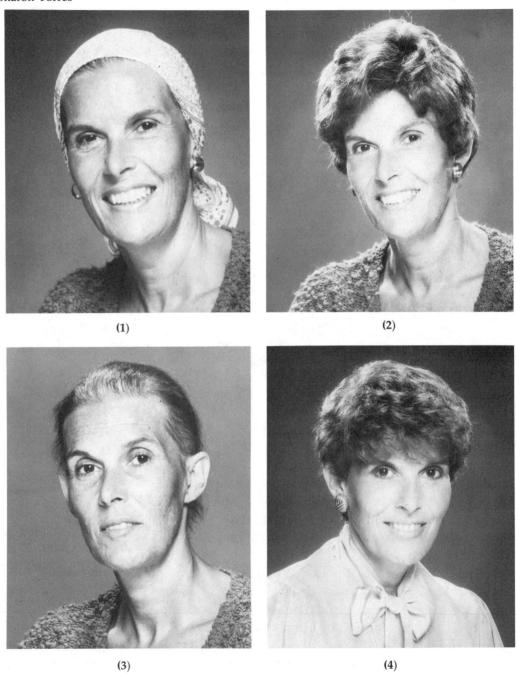

(1)

(2)

(3)

(4)

Sharon Torres

"I'm pretty happy with my scarf," Sharon confessed when I first discussed the possibility of a makeover with her. But she agreed to bring in her wig and her big brown eyes for a few hours with the beauty experts.

Sharon had lost about 75 percent of her hair during three and a half months of chemotherapy. She bought a wig before she began chemo but never felt entirely comfortable with it. "It wasn't the real me," she said. "I felt artificial and foolish in it." In fact, Sharon went so far as to admit that she hated her wig. And she had the usual complaints—it was tight and it was hot.

Photo 1: Sharon arrived in her everyday look—with a scarf coordinated to her outfit and a pair of earrings. "I bought a wardrobe of scarves which I wore in a lot of different styles and felt very comfortable in," she said.

Photo 2: Sharon put on the hated wig and we all knew why she hated it—it looked "wiggy."

Photo 3: Sharon without wig, scarf, or makeup. Eyelashes have thinned out from chemo; about 25 percent of her own hair remains.

Photo 4: The "new" Sharon Torres emerges after a session with Marilyn and Josef. "Do I get to keep the wig?" was the first thing she asked after the makeover was complete. (She wore it home and quit wearing her scarves!)

Jane Shimizu

"I've just dumped my wig, but I don't know what to do with my hair," explained Jane Shimizu when approached for a makeover. Jane's last chemo treatment had been six months before; since then she had had dual breast implants. She was anxious to begin her new life with a touch of glamour. "I didn't realize the extent of my vanity regarding my hair, so it was far more devastating than losing my breasts when my hair fell out. I got over it and wore a wig all the time. I enjoyed the wig after I overcame the idea that I needed to wear it."

Jane Shimizu

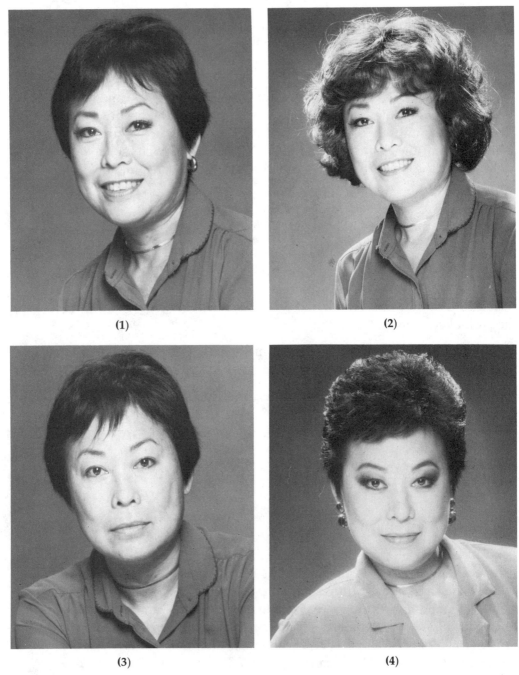

(1)   (2)

(3)   (4)

Photo 1: Jane arrived at the studio with her pixie hairstyle. Her hair had hardly been touched since chemo, except that occasional longer strands had been trimmed off when they got in the way. Jane does her hair color herself and had already given herself a shampoo-in color treatment to cover gray. Jane wore false eyelashes to fill out her thinner lashes.

Photo 2: Jane's BW turned out to be one of her least favorite wigs. She had finally settled on a longer, fuller, curlier style that reached to her shoulders. But she let us take a look at her BW, so that everyone would know that you have a lot of choices and that it's not a big deal if after you've bought one wig, you find another that you like better.

Photo 3: Jane au naturel.

Photo 4: Although Sachi trimmed off over 25 percent of her newly won locks, Jane wasn't complaining. Sachi pronounced her hair in good condition and plenty thick before she trimmed it to a fashionable bob. "I just love it!" said Jane. She is sans false eyelashes as well.

Karen Luce

Karen Luce agreed to be made over so that people could appreciate the versatility a totally bald head offers. She is not a cancer patient but suffers from a disease called alopecia universalis—for one reason or another, all the hair on her body has fallen out. It may grow back again and it may not—no one really knows. In the meantime, Karen has adjusted and now helps other women who suffer from hair loss—be it from alopecia or cancer—deal with the experience. "It's a part of your body that you lose, and you have to grieve for it; you have to come to grips with it," she advises. "When it first happened to me, I couldn't believe it. My hair was me, it was everything I was—it defined my femininity, my sexuality. Now I know that bald is beautiful, and I ask other women to take some time out to really think about themselves and their priorities. If you relax about it, you can have some fun with wigs and with being bald. Your attitude will make or break you. Sure, you'll get moments when you wonder what you ever did to deserve this, when you realize how unfair it is—but when you're alive and-

Karen Luce

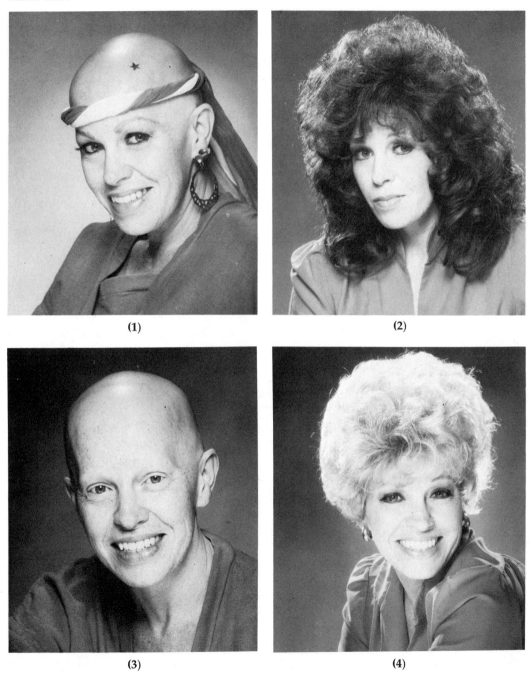

(1)

(2)

(3)

(4)

healthy, you know what's really important. Life is too short to spend it worrying about what you cannot change."

Photo 1: Karen's trademark look—her totally bald pate, a headband, and a star. Her eyebrows were drawn on with pencil; she wore false eyelashes.

Photo 2: Karen in one of her many wigs. Her skin tone allows her a wide range of color choices, which she takes advantage of. It's not unusual for Karen to be a blond one day and a redhead the next.

Photo 3: The naked truth—no brows, no lashes, no nothing.

Photo 4: Josef felt that Karen's face could carry the drama of a big wig, so he decked her out movie-star-style with one of the Eva Gabor Dahling wigs, from the professional line. These wigs are available only through studios and wig specialists.

Geraldine Connor

Geri Connor had been living life as a blond—her medium-brown hair had been frosted for as long as she could remember, and she thought of herself as a blond. She wore a blond wig during chemotherapy, but panicked when her hair started to grow in—the doctor told her no hair color for a while.

"My hair grows while you watch it," Geri crowed with pride as she talked about the five months since her last chemo treatment, "but I wish it would get thicker!" Always plagued by thin hair, Geri saw so much daily change that she kept her spirits up by watching her hair fill in. But she needed a good transitional look.

Photo 1: Geri walked in the door—no wig. She hadn't had a haircut since the end of chemo. Look at all that virgin hair!

Photo 2: Geri in one of her several wigs—a blond bombshell.

Photo 3: Without makeup.

Photo 4: Sachi layered Geri's hair to give it more body and advised her

Geraldine Connor

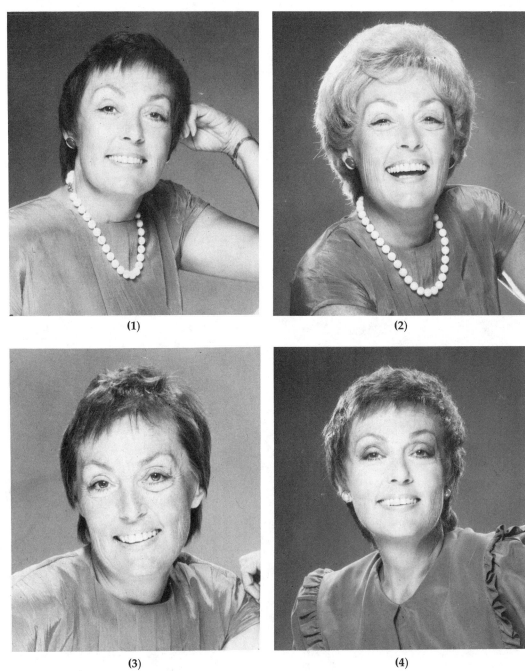

(1)

(2)

(3)

(4)

to forget about a perm for a while since her hair was changing so much. "Wait and see" is the best attitude during a period of great change, said Sachi. She also suggested that Geri ask her doctor if she could use Cellophanes, a brand of natural hair color that would brighten Geri's existing color and make the hair a bit thicker.

You in Transition

This is a fact of life: sick people look sick.

You cannot expect to look like your "old" self while you are ill or undergoing chemotherapy. There is every chance to believe, however, that you will return to your "old" self when treatment is finished. If you have trouble believing this, take a look at some of the women featured in this book—all, except one, cancer patients—or ask your oncologist to suggest a few former patients whom you can talk to. You will look fabulous again.

Your goal now is to look the best you can and not make yourself nuts worrying about it.

Your life changes when you become a cancer patient; you must expect your looks to change as well. Your body may or may not change, depending on surgery. Your face can change to reflect the condition of your health, the stress of your current situation, or weight loss or gain. You do yourself a terrible disservice if you think that you will not change. Accept change as inevitable and learn to live with it; accept the terms of your current situation and then fight back where it makes sense. A few wrinkles are meaningless in a fight of life over death.

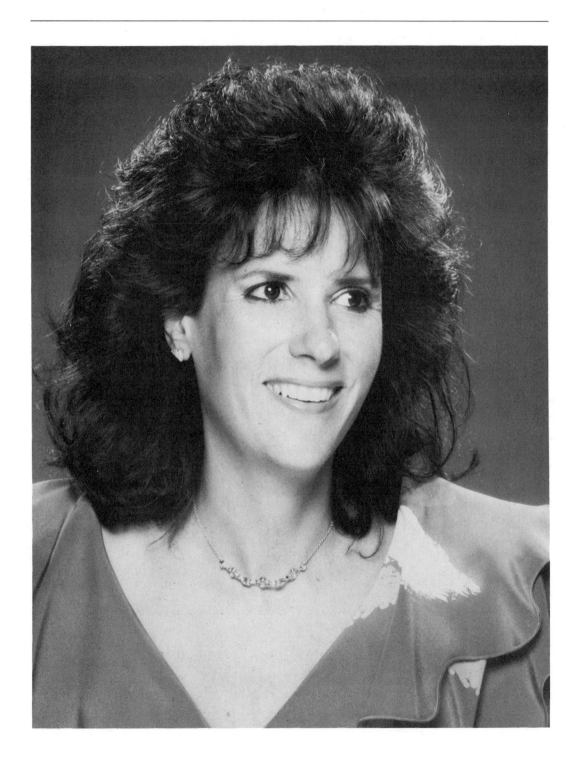

Chapter Five

Body Talk

Eyes

Visible Differences

The eyes are the focal point of a person's face cosmetically and the focal point of her world. Through our eyes we gain a large percentage of the information that leads us to form opinions and make judgments. The eyes are also basic to our communication with others. Without our eyes, how could musicians and rock-and-roll stars get rich with tunes like "Jeepers Creepers! Where'd Ya Get Those Peepers?" "Bette Davis Eyes," and "The Eyes of Texas Are upon You"?

The eye is a spherical structure known to doctors as the "globe." The outermost layer of the eye includes what we normally refer to as the "white" part (the *sclera*) and a clear part that covers the *iris* (colored part), called the *cornea*. The second layer of the eye includes the colored part (iris) and the rest of the interior structure, which is the *choroid*— a part of the eye that can become malignant. The third and innermost layer of the eye holds the *retina*, which contains the actual machinery (you remember those rods and cones from sixth-grade science) that bounces the image you see to your brain. Although cancer of the eye is not very common, it is possible. If you have cancer in part of your eye, these terms will soon become part of your everyday language.

Surrounding the eye are what are known as the accessory structures of the eye. You and I call them eyelids. The main jobs of the eyelids are to protect the eye—from both light and debris—and to make and distribute tears. Environmental hazards (smog and the like) also affect the eyes. Blinking is a reflex action that occurs spontaneously about twenty-five times a minute—when you are awake, of course. There are also lots of little glands and ducts in the area surrounding the eye, all with the same job of protecting it so that you can see and live life without an eye infection. If you've ever had pinkeye, you can appreciate these little glands and ducts.

Eye Problems

Although it is possible to get cancer in the eye itself, eye cancer is rare in adults. The more common form of cancer to affect the eye is simple skin cancer (basal or squamus), which, when not arrested, can eat into the glands and ducts that protect the eye, work its way into the nose or sinuses, and gnaw right on through to the brain. Not a pretty picture—but an entirely preventable one.

When spotted in the early stages, skin cancers in the eye area do not pose a serious threat either to your health or to your appearance. The key, of course, is to discover the cancer before it gets to the duct areas. Because skin cancer in this area is relatively slow-growing, an annual eye checkup should keep you protected from further hazard. If, however, you spot any of the warning signs of skin cancer, see your ophthalmologist as soon as possible.

Skin cancer near the eye is not a secondary symptom caused by regular radiation treatment or chemotherapy. Although some skin cancers result from toxic levels of chemicals used in polycytoxic chemo, the eye and the skin surrounding it are not usually affected by these drugs. About the only side effect a chemo patient may have that relates specifically to the eyes is dryness and redness—this may cause irritation for contact lens wearers.

The most common place near the eye for skin cancer to appear is on the lower lid, right where the sun is likely to hit it. In fact, over 50 percent of all skin cancers in the eye area are located on the lower lid. The type of treatment depends on the exact location of the tumor and its size. There are three basic alternatives: (1) surgery, (2) freezing, and (3) radiation.

Surgery: Surgery is often the choice for skin cancers around the eye-because the scars can easily be hidden in the normal folds of the skin. A plastic surgeon can even "fix" your eyelids at the same time. For the patient with recurring cancers in this area, repeated surgery is not recommended, because of the cumulative scar tissue.

Freezing (Cryotherapy): Freezing has proved to be an excellent method for destroying cancer cells. Cancer cells die faster than normal cells because they metabolize faster; freezing offers a good chance of killing off the bad guys in one blast. There's even more good news about the freezing process—it does not harm the tear ducts and though eyes will appear swollen for three to six months after treatment, they will return to their normal appearance. The bad news? Freezing permanently destroys the eyelashes in the area that has been treated and also causes depigmentation of the skin.

Radiation: Patients are fitted with a lead contact lens (painlessly inserted with a local anesthetic) before they get zapped. Radiation works quite well and side effects are minimal; the skin around the eyes may lose pigment and become lighter than the rest of the skin in that area, a slight cosmetic problem that can be corrected with makeup. Lashes will be permanently lost. The tear duct may also be destroyed in treatment, which will cause a person to have runny eyes. Luckily, a prosthetic tear duct (a Jones' Tube) can usually be constructed to solve this problem.

Cancer of the eyeball (globe) may be treated with either radiation or surgery; although immunotherapy has been discussed, it is still in the experimental stages and is not yet considered an acceptable method of treatment. Polycytoxic chemotherapy is used to treat one or two types of cancer affecting this part of the eye.

One of the newest methods of treatment involves the implantation in the eye of tiny radioactive seeds. Eyes will become reddened and swollen during this treatment, but will return to normal several weeks after the removal of the seeds. Under inspection, there will be no discernible difference in your eye after treatment. The technique of interstitial implants is becoming more and more refined and yielding increasingly better results every year.

LOOKING OUT FOR TROUBLE

As with all cancers, early detection is the best weapon we have. An annual checkup with an ophthalmologist (a medical doctor, as opposed to an optometrist, who is not) is a must. Keeping a Baseline Beauty Profile (see Chapter One) is also a good idea, especially if you have moles, pigment, or growths on your face in the area near your eyes. Also be on the lookout for these symptoms of eye cancer:

- One eye (usually not both) bulges. It will be easy for you or a friend to notice this discrepancy because your two eyes will look different. Each side may appear perfectly normal, but *together* they will look wrong.

- A change in the pupil. The pupil (the black center circle) is larger in the affected eye than in the nonaffected eye. This is most easily noticed in light-colored eyes. The pupil may also be irregular in shape.

- The eyes may not move together, or one eye may not move as far as the other.

- An eyelid may droop, or the blink rate in one eye may be different from that of the other.

- Watering or redness may show up early. This symptom will very much resemble pinkeye, and the doctor may actually treat you for pinkeye before the cancer is discovered.

- Double vision. Talk to your doctor.

Because many of the symptoms of eye cancer resemble those of other eye disorders, you need to have an excellent ophthalmologist and an attentive mind. If you notice changes in your condition, report them, don't ignore them.

DRY EYES

Dry eyes are usually not a symptom of cancer but a side effect of treatment. Although each person's eyes have a different amount of fluid, most people complain about some amount of dryness in their eyes while they are undergoing chemotherapy. The problem usually manifests itself first among contact lens wearers, who will suddenly find that their lenses feel tight or scratchy. Any of the many types of artificial tears on the market may help alleviate the discomfort. Many chemo patients who normally wear contacts say they prefer not to wear the lenses on the day of treatment and the day or so after, mostly because they know they will be sick and find the lenses just one extra thing to care for. If you are one of those lens wearers who does not even own a pair of glasses, get a pair made up at the time you begin chemotherapy. You might never see as well with glasses as you do with lenses, but you'll be buying yourself a lot of convenience. With discount and designer-style eyeglasses now available in almost every city, there's no reason not to have at least one pair of glasses at your immediate disposal.

If you find your eyes stinging or burning, you may be suffering from dry eyes. If artificial tears in a bottle are not convenient for you to use (you sometimes have to apply them as frequently as every hour), you may want to ask your doctor about Lacrisert, a solid particle of liquid that can be inserted into the eye. It's the size and shape of half a grain of rice and it slowly dissolves in the eye, offering extra moisture over a period of eight to ten hours. Some people adore the ease of the insert; others find it feels as if they have something in their eye.

For those whose eyes are so dry that the eye movement during sleep causes irritation or even abrasion of the cornea, a lubricating ointment such as Lacri-Lube may be applied at bedtime. There are also prescription drops that stimulate the lacrimal glands to produce more tears. Warm compresses will help stimulate the glands as well.

If all else fails, peel an onion.

Rubbing dry eyes can lead to infection; don't be embarrassed to ask your doctor about a fix—before you have a serious problem.

Eyebrows and Eyelashes

Some of the patients who lose their body hair as a result of chemotherapy also lose their eyebrows and eyelashes. Some lose just their eyebrows and *not* their eyelashes. If the hair loss is drug-induced, the brows and lashes will return when body hair returns—about six weeks after cessation of treatment.

If eyebrows and lashes are lost as a result of radiation of the eye area, they are unlikely to grow back. If you have this problem, you have several choices:

- You can get an eyebrow transplant.

- You can use theatrical eyebrows.

- You can draw eyebrows on with pencil.

- You can use artificial eyelashes.

- You can have eyelashes from another part of the eye moved.

Eyebrows

The human face looks empty without eyebrows; most patients who have lost them feel the need to define their eyes with some type of brow. Even men who are comfortable with bald pates during chemo can feel uncomfortable without brows. The dictates of recent fashion have made it acceptable for men to have heavy brows, while women's brows are to be thinner, finer, and better defined. Thus, more men use theatrical eyebrows and more women use eyebrow pencil.

Theatrical eyebrows are available through beauty supply stores, wig dealers, and some custom outlets. Essentially they are a series of hairs attached to a fine-mesh net. You stick the net to your skin with spirit gum. The oilier your skin, the more trouble you will have in getting the brows to stay on. Most people do tolerate them, however.

If your eyebrows are gone forever, you might consider a transplant, although currently only about 10 percent of the eligible patients choose this alternative. A transplant is not a difficult operation—a small section of scalp hair is taken from the back of the head and transplanted to the brow area by a plastic surgeon. There is one small catch—the new brows grow just like the hair on your head—you'll have to trim them to keep them in shape. And don't pluck, since you won't get new ones.

For drawing on eyebrows, the easiest technique is to use several soft feather strokes, rather than to try to draw one continuous line and then fill it in—unless you're anxious to look like Greta Garbo. The trick to drawn-on brows is not how you draw them, but that the two *match* so that you don't look cockeyed. Luckily, the follicles of your original brows will have left little marks in your skin: they are your best guideline. Over a period of years, these dots will disappear, but if your eyebrow loss is temporary, you'll have no trouble. Although it was once popular for women to shave off their brows and then draw in new ones at a higher plateau than their original ones, this is not a particularly natural style and probably won't give you much satisfaction.

Eyelashes

There was a time in American (and British) fashion history when an attractive young woman could not consider leaving the house without at least one row of false eyelashes attached to her lids. Three pairs (two upper, one lower) were not uncommon. Although the big-eye look has been replaced by a more natural look, false eyelashes are a welcome tool for those women who lose their lashes to radiation or chemotherapy. (For whatever reason, few men use false lashes.)

Applying false eyelashes is a matter of dexterity and practice. You cannot expect to apply them perfectly the first time, nor can you expect that once you get the hang of it you will always achieve perfection in sixty seconds flat. It takes time and care to apply the lashes; you cannot rush the process. Old hands at it give themselves four or five minutes for both eyes; when you are first beginning it may take you as long as fifteen minutes for both eyes. If you allow yourself the time in your schedule, you won't feel pressured and sabotage the results or give up in despair.

If you have always considered yourself a cosmetic klutz, you should consult a beauty expert or cosmetologist about false eyelashes. Let the expert choose the lashes, trim them, fit them, and then teach you how to apply them. This should not be an expensive procedure. If you have more confidence, you may want to do all this on your own; it's not hard.

1. Eyelashes are available in discount health and beauty stores and need not be expensive to be satisfactory. They are easily lost or destroyed, so do not invest a lot of money. In the late 1960s you could get a fine pair of eyelashes for $1; now you can get a good pair for $2.50. Although you can find lashes for $15 to $20, it is not necessary to pay this much.

2. Buy as natural a style as you can. No one's lashes should look like a caterpillar. Unless you are planning to perform *Aïda* at your next public appearance, buy a set of upper lashes (brown or black) that are not too thick. Buy "feathered" lashes whenever possible. This means the ends vary in length.

3. Fit the lash, without gluing it, to your eyelid to get the proper length; trim it to size with a small scissors. Fit each eye individually; it's not unusual for your eyes to differ slightly in size.

4. Once the lashes are the right length horizontally, feather the hairs with your small scissors by cutting them at an angle. Remember that the outer end should be longer than the inner. Look at some real lashes and judge accordingly. Do not exceed normal length unless you want to look like Endora on *Bewitched*.

5. Use an eyelash adhesive and not a household glue. If you get an allergic reaction, try another brand. Apply a thin stream of the adhesive to the band of the lash. Do not apply adhesive to your skin. Allow the adhesive to sit on the lash band for a few seconds, to get "tacky," as they say in the glue business. Then apply the lash to your lid.

6. Applying the lash to the lid does take some practice. It's natural for you to be nervous for this part, but calm down. Practice is all it takes to perfect this technical skill. Aim to place the midpoint of the lash band close to your natural lash line, at the midpoint of your lid. This should be your first contact point. Wait half a second, maybe a full second, and then touch the outer part of the lash to your skin; the outer part is easier than the inner because the hairs are longer. Finally, attach the inner corner. Some women use an unsharpened pencil, an orange stick, or the blunt end of their tweezers to gently tap the lash band in place on the lid. You certainly don't want to poke yourself in the eye, but some kind of pressure on the band

usually helps it adhere to the lid better. If the lashes have slipped upward, the pressure can be applied in a downward motion that brings the lashes to rest in the proper place. This, again, is a matter of practice. If you are right-handed, you'll find the right eye is easier to apply than the left. Do the more difficult eye first, since you will need more patience. Using an illuminated magnifying mirror may help people who use reading glasses.

7. Give the lashes a few seconds to settle down on your lids. You may then apply mascara if desired. Mascara probably isn't needed, but the additional touch of mascara glumped onto lashes will make you look more natural.

Lashes may also be applied to the lower lids, although you may find that makeup does just as well and that the lower lids are not worth the trouble of additional lashes. There are two good makeup tricks for the lower lid: a band of eyeliner (you may want to consider permanent eyeliner, which your doctor applies in tattoo form—see discussion below) or a series of vertical lines that stimulate lashes and fool anyone who is not nose-to-nose with you. If this trick sounds ridiculous, please rethink it: Mary Quant invented it in the big-eye days of the late 1960s, and it was considered the de rigueur method of enhancement by models of the time. (Some used false lashes and *then* filled in with the vertical lines!) If you have the patience of a saint, you can apply lower lashes either individually or in tiny clumps. Be sure to use an eyeliner after applying them, so that they look like a cohesive unit, rather than like a few dumb clumps of eyelashes in the middle of nowhere.

"I thought that not having eyelashes would be the worst thing in the world," says one woman. "I mean the worst thing after, you know, the worst thing. Every time I looked in the mirror, I had to look twice because my face looked so washed out, so strange. But what's so funny about it is that after a while, it just didn't matter. I wear false eyelashes on the top, and I just let the bottom go with a little bit of eyeliner. I don't think anyone can tell the difference anyway. I was never one of those women with thick, long eyelashes. You know, I think men get the good eyelashes anyway. Mine were always breaking off, and I never knew if I should use mascara or if that would make it worse—and now, who cares?"

LASH TRANSFER

If a small portion of each lash has been destroyed by radiotherapy but the rest of it remains healthy and intact, a plastic surgeon can perform a lash transfer. Lash hairs from another part of the eyelid are simply grafted into the "bald" space, filling it out and making the loss less noticeable. Because the new lashes are taken from the corners of the eye, their loss is not as conspicuous. Your eyes can be made to match. This procedure is relatively simple; it can be done in an office visit.

Only about 5 percent of the patients who qualify for this surgery take advantage of it. Why? The loss of a few lashes doesn't really mean much to them. They manage quite well with false eyelashes or without artifice and see no reason to undergo more surgery.

PIGMENT TATTOO

You've heard about it and probably laughed about it. Permanent eyeliner, which is actually a pigment tattoo applied to the upper and lower lids, began in California as one of those wacky fads that has ended up as a mainstream treatment.

Several companies now provide training, equipment, and dye to ophthalmologists who perform this service, which many doctors recommend to chemotherapy patients who have lost their eyelashes.

A simple in-office procedure, pigment tattooing is done with a wand that looks like a white candle attached to a geiger counter. The machine makes a dull hum while the doctor applies a series of dots to the lashline, using the dye shade of choice (brown, black, gray, or brown-black). The dye spreads upon contact with the skin, so the tiny dots appear to be one thin line of color. The process takes about twenty to thirty minutes and costs $800 to $1000. This tattoo is as permanent as the one of the naked dancing lady.

Because the tattoo gives an outline and definition to the eyes, it is often suggested to patients who have lost lashes. Many doctors add the tattoo after rebuilding the eyelids or performing facial reconstruction, although the area must be totally healed before the tattoo can be applied.

Eye Tricks

If you've had eye surgery, facial reconstruction, dry or tired eyes from chemo, or simply a bad day, you may want to try some of these tricks:

- For dry or tired eyes, apply an ice pack and take a break in which you raise your head higher than your feet. Indulge in one of those plastic eye masks that contain a gel which can be refrigerated or frozen. There are even masks that cover the entire face.

- If complications from chemo are causing puffiness in the eye area, again, try the eye mask. Also, sleep with the head of the bed elevated so that the head is higher than the feet. If you can learn to sleep sitting up with your head resting on a layer of three or four pillows, much of the puffiness may subside.

- If your contact lenses are bothering you, but you are reluctant to switch to glasses, ask your doctor about some of the newer types of lenses that are designed for dry eyes. Remember that they may not work for you during this period of your life, but if you are determined, don't be discouraged from trying.

- If surgery has left you with one eye that is smaller than the other, ask your doctor to prescribe a pair of glasses with a lens made to "distort" the image of the eye to the "right" size. We all know that some glasses make the eyes appear bigger and some can make them appear smaller. A tricky doctor can use one of these lenses to fool the outside world into thinking your eyes are the same size. Then he will prescribe a contact lens or a refraction for the eyeglass lens that will counter any visual distortion the lens may cause.

- In some cases where the surface of the eye is discolored or cosmetically damaged, a contact lens can be worn to make the eye appear totally "normal."

- If your eyes just don't "look right" cosmetically, consider a pair of glasses—even if you don't need them—to shift the focal point of your face away from your eyes. Glasses have become such a fashion accessory that no one considers them unattractive any more. A lens with a slight tint, or a gradient tint, may be just the camouflage you need to hide a not quite perfect eye. "Often doctors can correct the problem to the 80 percent mark," says Dr. William Fein, an ophthalmologist–plastic surgeon. "Then we need a little camouflage to go the tiny extra bit of the way."

Lungs

Although lung cancer is an internal disease that does not cause obvious cosmetic problems, the removal of a lung, or any type of chest surgery, can cause scar damage.

"I got home from the hospital and my mother was in the kitchen making me a cup of tea. I'm divorced, so my mother was helping me out. I was real weak, but getting better. Before I got into bed, when I was about to put on a nightgown, I looked at myself in the mirror and tears of self-pity just gushed out of my eyes. The scar was huge; of course, it was red and there were still stitches and it was the ugliest thing I'd ever seen. I kept thinking that no man would ever want to touch me again. I thought it was awful, and I didn't even feel glad to be alive. I got into bed, feeling really sorry for myself, and thought about my image in the mirror. I realized I had two breasts—two very fine, healthy breasts. Once I put it in that perspective, I never felt sorry for myself again. In time, of course, the scar healed up, and it's not much of anything any more."

The type of surgery your doctor performs depends on the site of the tumor (right lung is more common than left) and the extent of metastasis. The doctor may remove part or all of one lung, or he may decide the case is inoperable and simply close up the chest. There are three major different types of lung cancer: squamous cell and adenocarcinoma, which are sometimes cured by surgery, and oat cell, which is usually not operated on.

Patients who are still upset about the aesthetics of their scar a year

after surgery should discuss collagen injections with a qualified dermatologist or plastic surgeon. Not all dermatologists are expert at the
use of collagen; not all doctors are in favor of the use of the product or
believe in its long-range effects. This bears careful investigation on
your part. You must have a tolerance test for collagen, which should
probably be performed early in your decision-making process, so that
you don't waste any more time, energy, or money on consultations if
you turn out to be ineligible for the procedure.

Head and Neck

Patients with cancer in the head and neck areas often worry about
scars, disfiguration, and life after surgery. Many worry that life will not
be worth living, even if they are cancer-free. They imagine with horror
that they will be freaks—that friends and family members will look
away or come up with excuses not to see them. They worry that they
will not be able to cope.

This is perhaps the hardest type of cancer to cope with because it is
so visible; yet the miracles now wrought by plastic surgeons and prosthetics makers are so impressive that even the Bionic Woman would be
awestruck. Some patients receive a prosthetic device at the time of the
original tumor surgery. Other patients heal from their primary surgery,
receive chemotherapy or radiotherapy, and then have additional surgery for cosmetic and psychological reasons. Still others are given prosthetic devices that fit onto the face—often with the aid of an attractive
pair of glasses—and make its contours appear as even and smooth as
they were prior to the discovery of the malignancy.

When you first learn you have cancer in this part of your body, you
may find yourself wishing for something simpler, like breast or colon
cancer—cursing your bad luck, beseeching God for a reason that this
happened to you. As you work through your anger, your readiness for
change will rise to the surface and you will slowly adapt and learn the
options that are open to you. Consult several experts, read up on the
advances being made. With today's technology, no one—man or
woman—need feel that he is a freak. Never have doctors been more

responsive to the cosmetic problems wrought by cancer of the head and neck, and never have there been so many possibilities.

Know your cosmetic and surgical options *before* surgery; know what improvements can be made *after* the initial surgery. A well-educated patient who is ready to learn and who is ready to grasp reality and see the excitement of the possibilities ahead will come out of this experience victorious.

If your surgery includes a tracheostomy, or installation of a "trach" (pronounced trake)—a breathing tube that is inserted in the trachea and that opens at the surface of your neck—do not attempt to cover the apparatus with makeup or camouflage. No throat creams over the trach, please. This practice could lead to infection or breathing complications.

It is acceptable, and advised, to cover the trach with a scarf or ascot made of light, porous material. This can be casually, yet artfully, tied to cover the opening without impeding your breathing. If you consider that diamonds are a girl's best friend, you might stop by Harry Winston jewelers in New York to see if they've got a diamond choker that will help your camouflage. Pearl chokers (ala Princess Di) and "dog collar" necklaces are also acceptable if they aren't too tight.

Just as "they" don't like to see women without hair, "they" are often upset by the sight of an open trach. Disguise is easy, rest assured. Any ostomy takes getting used to, but with time and patience you will learn to live with yours. It beats the alternative.

Hands and Nails

Hands

Unless you have a tumor on one of them, your hands will be affected by treatment in a nonspecific manner, if at all.

With some patients on some drugs (not all patients, not all drugs), it is relatively common to have itching of the palms, tingling in the hands, sweaty or clammy hands, or even a rash. The rash may be just on the palms, or it may be on the whole hand. It may even be on one hand and not the other.

For most patients, the hands remain unaffected and can become a source of pleasure. At a time when your body image may have to be rebuilt, it's nice to take comfort in a beautiful pair of hands. Buy yourself a new bottle of nail polish and enjoy. If you get blue about your wig or your dry skin, glance down at your nails and smile.

Nails

The nails are miniature plates that grow out from under the cuticle. The hidden part is alive; the emerging fingernail is not. Nails are made of keratin, just like hair; therefore, the same things that affect hair growth also affect nails. Eating well influences hair and nail health; chemotherapy affects hair more harshly than it does nails, but it still affects the nails.

The nail, constructed of three translucent layers, fits on top of a nail bed, which is also called the *quick*. At the finger end of the nail is the *lunula*, what we commonly refer to as the "moon." Around the margin of the nail bed is a horny type of skin, a toughened layer of the epidermis called the *cuticle*.

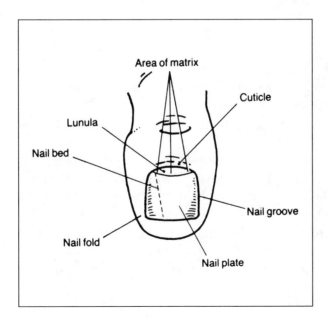

Although the fingernails are more often affected by chemo than the rest of the hand, the side effects do not usually preclude a manicure. Dry, brittle nails are common to chemo patients; weakness and flakiness are not unusual; stripes, color bands, or even discoloration of nails can occur. If your nails turn slightly yellow, don't worry about it. Cover them with polish. You may buy nail bleach at a beauty supply store, but it will not work very well since the source of the discoloration is within your own body. Grin and bear it.

The nail bed and the bottom layer of the nail have a rich blood supply. It is through this supply that the effects of chemotherapy are carried to your nails. But nails, unlike hair, keep on growing at a steady rate—they do not have a resting period. The right hand's nails grow slightly faster than those of the left. Age and sex do not affect growth. Growth rate may actually be higher with some diseases and is sometimes lower as a result of chemotherapy. Although doctors say they have no substantial medical evidence that gelatin tablets increase the growth rate or the strength of nails, many cosmetologists recommend these tablets specifically to chemo patients. A dose of anywhere from 2 to 7 grams of gelatin a day will not hurt you and may help your nails through the difficulties of chemotherapy. Expect no miracles.

If you are a person who regularly has a professional manicure, you may continue to do so now. *But do not have your cuticles cut.* If your white blood count is 1000 or lower, it is dangerous to have your cuticles cut because of the possibility of infection. If your white blood count is over 1000, ask your doctor if he recommends cutting. Cuticle creams will usually do the trick without a scissors anyway; many cosmetologists are opposed to cutting.

If you want to give yourself a manicure, follow these easy steps:

1. Remove nail polish twenty-four hours prior to your manicure. Use a gentle nail polish remover that is oil-based. Nail polish remover is potentially damaging to healthy nails; it can be especially drying during chemotherapy. Ask your beauty supply shop about cream polish removers—they exist. Because they are lanolin-based, they will protect your nails more. Remember, they don't work as fast as the old-fashioned method. Be patient; allow some extra time and keep your nails healthy longer. Rinse your hands thoroughly after using nail polish remover, and moisturize them with lotion.

2. Inspect your nails for significant changes; if you find any, record them in your Baseline Beauty Profile (Chapter One). If you notice the nail curving into the nail bed, do not proceed with the manicure until you've reported to your doctor.

3. Get out all your supplies. Set yourself in a comfortable position where you can relax for at least an hour. Use a lap board if your manicure site is in bed.

4. Begin your manicure by soaking your nails, one hand at a time, in a bowl of warm water mixed with baby oil. Soak for one to two minutes.

5. Dry your hands on a towel, using the terry cloth to push back the cuticles gently.

6. Apply cuticle cream as per directions on the package, allowing it to set on your hands for a minute or two. Cuticle cream and cuticle removers are alkaline materials in cream or liquid form. They do not actually gobble up your cuticle in order to remove it; they soften the horny layer of epidermis to make it more malleable. Now, using an orange stick that is lavishly wrapped in cotton, push back your cuticles. Be very careful not to tear or break your skin.

7. Rinse off the cuticle cream. Dry your hands and apply hand cream and/or lotion all the way up to the elbows. Apply oil to your nails and the cuticles surrounding them. You may use Crisco, olive oil, baby oil, eye cream, or any other emollient cream or oil. Massage each nail as you rub in the goo. Relax for five minutes to allow your skin to absorb the cream.

8. File your nails with an emery board, not a nail file. Go in one direction only and gently shape them. It is more difficult to file nails that have already been moisturized, but this method is safer for the chemo nail. If you find you are too greasy even to manage a nail file, rinse your hands very quickly and pat them dry. Then file.

9. If any break in a nail extends below the quick, discontinue the manicure process for that nail. Under no circumstances should you apply glue to the nail to mend the break. Bandage the nail until it grows out to a point where it can be cut off without danger of infection. Watch the tear for color changes; report any to your doctor.

10. Do not buff your nails.

11. Apply a base coat. The kind with fibers is great if your nails are weak.

12. Top the base coat (with fibers) with ridge filler. This flattens the fibers so that they don't stick up in the polish.

13. Apply nail polish. If you aren't handy with the traditional polish, get one of the new pen-style polish brushes. You don't have to worry about spilling these; they're great for hospital visits and in-bed manicures.

14. Apply a second coat of polish.

15. Finish with a top coat, preferably an acrylic one.

16. Allow the nails to dry thoroughly. Allow one hour for relaxing and drying.

Nail- and hand-care products have proliferated lately, but the best place to find a good selection of them is still a beauty supply store. Barielle, a nail-strengthening cream that is sold in department stores (and is rather pricey) gets good grades from patients and nonpatients. Mavala of Switzerland also sells a complete line of over one dozen nail-care products, also available in department stores.

Some tips:

- Since you will be moisturizing your body regularly, be sure to lavish cream or lotion on your hands whenever possible.

- At bedtime, put a dab of cream on each fingernail and massage it in a circular pattern, working your way to the cuticles. Push back the cuticles at the base of each nail with a towel or thumb. Be careful not to tear the skin.

Although having your nails professionally "wrapped" will keep them strong during chemo, this is a costly and time-consuming process: a manicurist will individually wrap each fingernail with silk, tissue paper, or another fiber and then cover it with glue, sealer, and polish. You can strengthen your own nails and get the same effect by using a fiber-weave base coat (about $3) under your polish. There are many brands available.

If you have never had nice nails, or if chemo demolishes your nails, fight back, with the understanding that this is a temporary condition. *Self* magazine recently conducted an experiment during which beginners grew a handsome set of nails merely by going off for a weekly manicure. If you can afford to do so, get a professional manicure. (Remember to tell the manicurist not to clip your cuticles!) If you can't afford a manicure, get a buddy and do each other's nails. Call a local beauty school and see if a student can help you. Your hospital or treatment center may also have a manicure program. (Don't laugh—many hospitals do. They admit to the therapeutic benefits of a manicure.)

If you are a chemo patient, *never bite your nails.*

Do not have plastic, acrylic, "Patty," or porcelain nails applied on top of your own nails while you are undergoing chemotherapy. If you already have them, discuss it with your doctor. Don't be surprised if they snap off easily during the treatment period.

FOR NAIL BITERS

People who bite their nails always mean to stop; they just can't get around to it. If you are a cancer patient who bites her nails, congratulations—today's the day to stop that gnawing. OK, OK, most nail biters chew their nails and cuticles out of nervous habit, and having cancer does indeed tend to make you nervous. Sure, biting your nails beats smoking and drinking, but for the patient about to undergo chemotherapy, nail biting can be just as hazardous to your health as these other vices.

Raw, ragged nails and open cuticles can become easily infected when your white blood count is low. If your doctor doesn't want a manicurist to properly trim dead skin by means of cuticle cutting, imagine what he thinks of nails that are bitten to the quick.

Use your postsurgery time to heal—let your surgical wound heal and your nails grow in. You don't need a set of claws that would make the emperor of China proud—just let the nails grow out past the quick. Get a professional manicure to help you through the first two weeks, which will be the hardest. If you can't afford a professional manicure (have at least one a week), find out if your hospital has a beauty program whereby you can get a free manicure. Especially if you are a nail biter, this is a medical problem now, not just a cosmetic one. Knit, keep your fingers busy, finger a rosary or some worry beads. Use foul-tasting polishes to help you quit biting. Now is the time.

Feet

As appendages, the hands and feet are pretty much a matched set. The feet are likely to react to chemo or radiation treatment in much the same way as the hands, although some people have reactions on one and not the other.

Don't be alarmed by flushed feet, tingling feet, rashes or bumps, peeling, or itching. Do report problems to your doctor and ask for treatment if relief is needed. If you suffer from athlete's foot, be sure to treat it immediately. When left unattended, athlete's foot can cause skin to fissure and break open. This is not good for the cancer patient. Athlete's foot is not a serious problem, but it must be treated so that it does not become one.

Some people report swollen ankles and sore feet—much like during pregnancy—as a side effect of chemo or radiation. If these occur take some time out each day to elevate your feet. Try getting your feet higher than your head for twenty minutes.

Wear only comfortable shoes.

Some patients lose sensation in their feet during their treatment. If you suffer from this problem, do not go barefoot, and take time each night to inspect your feet. It's very possible for you to injure a foot without noticing it, and a cut could pose a problem if not handled properly. While this is not a common problem, it does affect some patients who take vincristine and *cis*-platinum. Diabetic patients may also have a loss of sensation in the feet.

Toenails

"My large toenails turned black during chemo, and one came off," reports one former patient. "They grew back, but they never grew back properly and are still a problem, two years later."

Check the color and condition of your toenails just as you do your fingernails. Note observations in the back of this book and report changes to your doctor.

THE DOCTOR'S APPROVED PEDICURE

The luxury of a pedicure is the rest, relaxation, and massage that goes with the polish. The polish is really secondary. Since it is very difficult to give yourself a relaxing pedicure because of the uncomfortable positions you have to assume, see if you can get someone in your family to help you out with this. You can even take turns treating each other. Patients have so many friends who ask, "What can I do?" This is something they can do for you! Just remember the two basic rules: don't *cut* the cuticles, and don't *cut* the toenail below the quick.

1. If you can afford it, buy yourself one of those electric foot-soaking machines. They cost about $20 at a discount appliance store. This is not a vibrator but a tub. Fill the tub with warm water, bubble bath, and baby oil. Do not use bath salts, because they are dehydrating. Turn on the machine, which will vibrate slightly, and enjoy the soak for fifteen minutes. If you think an electric foot-soaking machine is a silly waste of money, you will do just fine with a pan or bucket of hot water. Consider using some of the plastic utensils the hospital gave you when you checked out; often these are the perfect size for foot soaking. Even though hot water does dry out the skin, you will not have a pedicure so frequently that it matters in the long run. (Once a month is plenty.) Indulge and enjoy.

2. After the soak, dry your feet well. Then massage-in a body cream or lotion. Splurge on the massage time. Allow at least five minutes. This is a nice pick-me-up for circulation and can be very soothing. Naturally, a massage is more relaxing if someone else is doing it to you, but don't rule out self-massage; it is not hard to do. Slather on lots of cream or lotion during the process. Johnson & Johnson baby cream is a good one, and so is Nivea. A cream will do a little bit better job than a lotion, just because it's thicker.

3. Wrap part of a towel around your index finger, and use this to push down the cuticle on your big toes while the feet are still damp from the lotion or cream. *Do not cut the cuticle.*

4. Pat the foot dry, making sure you're not dripping with cream, oil, or lotion. Since many patients feel weak during treatment, be careful not to make yourself greasy or the floor slippery without a helping hand nearby.

5. Use blunt-edged baby scissors to cut your toenails. A clipper often cuts lower than intended. Trim the nail straight across the top; do not curve at the sides. While you are cutting, check each nail carefully. Make mental notes of the color and the growth pattern. It's not unusual for toenails to turn colors, become partially discolored or striped, or fall off. Still, any such change should be written down and reported to your doctor.

6. If you have any blisters or sores on your feet, note and keep an eye on them. Blisters should not be opened, because of the possibility of infection. Open sores should not be covered with lotions or creams and should be reported to your doctor. (*Note:* If you have open sores, get your doctor's permission *before* you have a pedicure. Soaking may be contraindicated.)

7. Finish off the pedicure with the application of polish. Wrap toilet paper in and out between your toes, or fit foam forms between them, to keep the nails apart. Apply base coat, color, and then top coat. Let dry thoroughly.

Teeth, Mouth, and Lips

Teeth

Doctors are still observing the effects of chemotherapy on teeth. Nothing *terrible* has happened to anyone, but change in color is not totally uncommon for some chemo and radiation patients. Mouth infections are common; discomfort with dentures is a possible problem.

Doctors consider it more important that their patients are free of other, unrelated dental problems, because once they are undergoing chemotherapy their white blood count becomes lowered and oral surgery for root-canal work or tooth removal is not recommended. Your doctor will usually suggest that you see your dentist for a checkup before you begin chemotherapy. Your dentist may want to consult with your oncologist before he begins any involved procedures.

DISCOLORATION

If you have a problem with tooth discoloration, talk to your dentist. Few patients complain of discolored teeth; those who do have the problem usually get it several years after chemo. If you find that the discoloration creates a cosmetic problem you can't live with, investigate these new techniques for brightening up that smile:

Bonding: Bonding has been used successfully for covering discoloration caused by antibiotics. It can also be used to fill in chipped, broken, or crooked teeth. The results are dramatic, fast, painless, and, well, expensive. Expect to pay $150 to $600 per tooth for the treatment. The more work per tooth, the higher the price. Bonding is believed to last three to eight years. Since it's a relatively new procedure, no long-range studies have been done. The dentist who performs the bonding will clean the teeth with an acid solution and then apply a resin on top of that. If the teeth are very dark, sometimes a lightener is applied before the resin. If you have treatment for color correction only, the teeth may have to be filed down after the resin has been applied. Bonding may not cover really dark spots and may make your "new" teeth look whiter than your untreated old ones. The bonding material may also crack or break off.

Bleaching: Bleaching counters mild discoloration but lightens all of the tooth, including the nondiscolored part. An oxidizing agent is used under heat or light for 20 to 40 minutes; the treatment is repeated several times, depending on the degree of the discoloration. Bleaching seems to last indefinitely; it is priced at $100 to $250 per treatment.

Painting: Tooth painting works well on slightly discolored teeth and is best done by a pro, although there are do-it-yourself kits. The price is about $150 per tooth. The painting requires skill, because the paint color should match your "normal" teeth as closely as possible. Painting doesn't last forever; it may chip or wear off.

Veneer: There are currently three different types of veneer being used: acrylic, resin, and porcelain. The veneer is custom-made from an imprint of the tooth; it is then coated with resin and attached to the tooth. Often the size of the tooth must be reduced slightly to accommodate the new front it receives. The cost is more or less equal to that of bonding, but the results and the life span of the treatment may be better.

Do not undergo any of these treatments without consulting your oncologist; make certain your dentist knows you have been a cancer patient.

DENTURES

If you have radiation to the mouth, you may find that your gums shrink. This will make your dentures uncomfortable and then unwearable. At the first sign of rubbing or discomfort, talk to your oral surgeon. It is very easy for the dentures to rub against your gums and cause sores, irritation, and eventual infection. If you notice a difference, mention it. Don't wait around for weeks to see if it will go away.

Patients who have no radiation to the mouth area but who have chemotherapy may also develop discomfort with dentures. This is less likely, but should be reported if the trouble persists over a forty-eight-hour period, to make sure there is no rubbing. Dryness in the mouth can be enough to cause discomfort with otherwise well-fitting dentures.

Mouth

While chemo affects the teeth of relatively few patients, many more people will complain of one or another small problem with their mouth. Some of the oral complications of chemotherapy include:

- Stomatitis (sores)

- Oral infections

- Dry, red, or rough lips

- Red, coated tongue

- Red, swollen gums

- White plaque

- Decreased saliva

- Difficulty in swallowing

- Mouth and tongue tenderness

Because any sores in the mouth have to be treated immediately, you should spend a few minutes a day, preferably in the morning and at night when the teeth are normally cleaned, for a quick oral self-examination.

1. Wash your hands thoroughly. You don't have to scrub like Dr. Kildare, but do have clean, dry hands.

2. Examine your mouth in front of a well-lighted mirror. If you do not have a makeup mirror with lights, you might consider buying one now.

3. Begin with the lips. They should be smooth and moist.

4. Next, look at your tongue. It should be moist, smooth, and pink.

5. Look under the tongue at the floor of the mouth—it, too, should be moist and pink.

6. Now, open your mouth as wide as you can and check the roof and the sides of the cheeks. They should be moist, pink, and free of spots or patches of color (dark or light).

7. Check the teeth. They should be white and without film.

Keeping your mouth healthy throughout chemo will keep down the number of complications you have, and make you feel as if you look better. Although few people will open your mouth and ask you to say "Ah," a mouth that feels fresh and clean has a good psychological effect.

As part of your twice-daily oral routine, after your mini-self-exam, follow these simple steps.

1. Clean your teeth with a soft toothbrush. Rinse thoroughly with water. Do not use an abrasive tooth powder. You may want to experiment with toothpaste for "sensitive" teeth, which is sold in grocery stores and drugstores, alongside regular toothpastes.

2. Forget your fancy-colored fast-lane mouthwash. Most commercial mouthwashes have alcohol in them and are dehydrating. A saline (salt water) gargle is your best bet (1 teaspoon salt to 1 quart water).

3. Use lip moisturizer constantly. Discuss the type with your physician. He may not want you to use petroleum jelly or mineral oil at night.

4. Use unwaxed dental floss every twenty-four hours—gently. If gums bleed, discontinue use. If gums continue to bleed off and on over a twenty-four-hour period, tell your doctor.

5. Report to your doctor any of the following: (a) difficulty in swallowing, (b) white patches in the mouth, (c) ulcerations, or (d) coating on the tongue.

DRY MOUTH

If you suffer from dry mouth, and most chemo patients do, there are a few methods for getting some relief—experiment a little until you find the best for you. Chew gum or keep hard candy available. There are many flavors of sugar-free candy; many patients swear by old-fashioned lemon drops or Life Savers. There are sucking candies with medication in them that are meant to stimulate saliva production. Carry a flask with you containing mouthwash for frequent refreshment stops. If you must use commercial mouthwash, dilute it at one part product to five parts water. This will give you a hint of the taste but not dry you out too much. Many patients report that they brush their teeth after each meal as a means of refreshing the mouth and keeping it moist. If you choose this method, avoid constant contact with the gums, which may be sore or tender during chemo and may therefore bleed more easily.

One good gargle for a sore mouth is a combination of salt and baking soda; another is one part peroxide to five parts water. This is for gargling only and should not be swallowed!

Lips

Everyone suffers from dry lips at one time or another—usually as fall turns to winter and the climate turns chilly. Although wintertime chapped lips may be annoying, they are not a serious problem. They are not a serious problem for cancer patients, either, but they do need a little more attention.

Dry lips are caused by changes in weather and/or changes in the air conditions around your lips; if you breathe out of your mouth, as many patients do (whether they have cancer or not), you will undoubtedly have parched lips. They can be uncomfortable, but they are problematic only if you bite at the skin or allow the dryness to lead to actual sores or cracks in the lips, since these leave the body open to infection.

Keeping your lips as smooth as possible will make you feel more glamorous and will eliminate the worry of infection. Begin your crusade for the lips as soon as you know that you are going to the hospital. You don't have to buy an expensive lip treatment—petroleum jelly will do just fine. If you find it too globby, try any of the ski products that come in tubes, or even a greasy type of lipstick that is laden with moisturizer. You don't have to get neurotic about it, but try to apply a protective coat whenever you think about it. Get a nurse or nurse's aide to help you, if you are too weak. A little bit of lipstick will help perk up your spirits while it protects your lips.

Your dry lips will heal automatically as you begin to recover from your surgery. Continue to baby them, however, especially if you are going to receive chemotherapy. Chemo is drying to all parts of the skin and especially affects the mucous membranes (such as those in your mouth)—so your lips will no doubt continue to feel parched. Keep them lubricated at all times; do not bite at them; don't lick them thinking your saliva will have a moisturizing effect (it won't—it only dries them out more). Report any open fissures to your doctor immediately.

Smoking

Needless to say, no cancer patient should smoke. If you insist on smoking, you may have more problems with dry mouth, tooth stains, and sores. If you have open lesions in your mouth, you must discontinue smoking at least until they heal.

Drinking

There are several reasons why excessive drinking is bad for your health. Even drinking in moderation may be troublesome for the patient undergoing chemotherapy. For one thing, liquor and wine leave a dry mouth, and a dry mouth that is getting even dryer is an uncomfortable mouth. You're better off with water or by remembering the five-to-one rule—mix five parts of water, seltzer, or mixer to every one part of wine or booze.

Oral Cancer

There is not a huge incidence of cases of oral cancer, but if you suffer from oral cancer, your concerns are very real.

Smoking is the number-one factor leading to oral cancer—and lung cancer as well. A recent study proves that women who smoke and drink may develop oral cancer as much as fifteen years earlier than the woman who does not smoke or drink! The cure rate for oral cancer is high when, as in other cancers, the malignancy is discovered early enough. Regular self-examination and consistent dental checkups are the best way to monitor the situation.

Consider any of these conditions as possible symptoms of oral cancer; see an oral surgeon immediately. Other physicians do not necessarily know much about the mouth or the beginnings of oral cancer;

and not all dentists are trained in the early detection of the disease. Report to your doctor:

- Sores that do not heal in two weeks

- Colored blotches in the mouth—red, white, or darkened

- Swelling or growths that do not diminish in one to two weeks

- Pain or loss of feeling in any part of the mouth

- Repeated bleeding for no apparent reason

Pain is not a necessary symptom. You can have oral cancer and feel absolutely nothing.

Treatment for oral cancer varies with the size and location of the tumor. The standard treatment has been surgery and radiotherapy, but new techniques are being tried, including cryosurgery (freezing), chemosurgery, and chemotherapy. The most exciting advance in the progress being made for head, neck, and oral cancer patients is that plastic and reconstructive surgeons now work with the oncological surgeon during the primary surgery, so that body parts can be reconstructed. The patient who fears disfigurement, or life behind a veil, will be pleased with the successes doctors now enjoy in restoring good looks and good health.

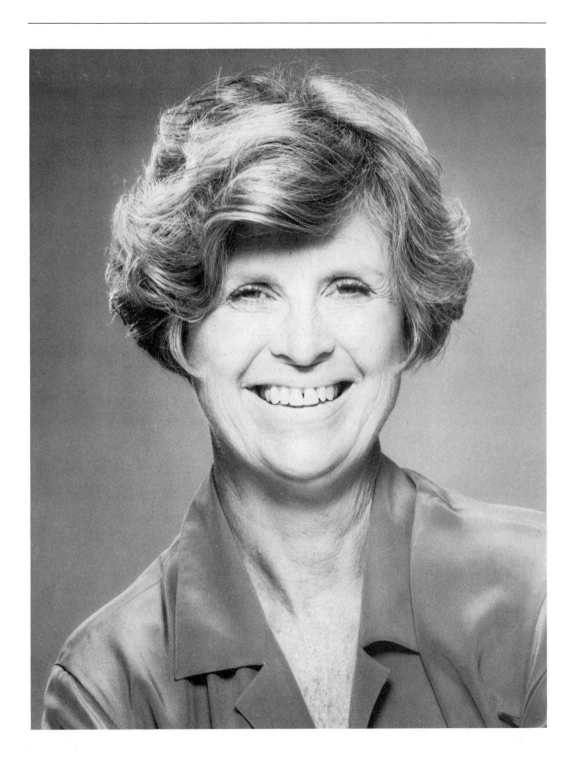

Chapter Six

PRIVATE TALK

The Unspeakable

Not long ago, it was considered impolite to say the word "breast"—or any of the scads of euphemisms—in mixed company. As recently as 1975, the word could not be used on television. Times, of course, have changed; men and women alike have become more comfortable talking about the more private body parts. With this ease—this nonchalance—has come the ability to also discuss cancer of the private parts. Breast cancer especially is now common luncheon and cocktail party chitchat; thanks to Ronald Reagan, one can even discuss colon cancer at the dinner table.

It is far less easy to discuss other private matters—such as stomas and ostomies, vulvectomies and vaginal reconstructions. Since bladder and bowel control will always be more personal subjects than breast care, it is natural enough that the subject is still somewhat of a social taboo. But with education and new understanding, the public will prove itself adaptable. As our willingness to discuss and to learn about the quality of life after private surgery increases, greater numbers of lives will be saved by a public that is willing to grasp the importance of early discovery.

Private matters are private, it's true. But the more people who learn that private cancers are not the end of the world, the more survivors we will have to share this world. It's worth it for all of us.

Breasts—Fear and More Fear

Nine-year-old Laura called her mother in sheer panic. Although it was four o'clock in the afternoon when Laura returned from school, and her mother would be home from work in less than two hours, Laura was very concerned about her health and her future. She had to talk to her mother immediately.

"Mother," she confided breathlessly, "I have a lump in my breast. Do you think I have cancer? Will my breast have to be cut off before it even starts to grow?"

Laura's mother does not have breast cancer and is not sure what conversation Laura overheard that brought her to such a state of alarm. Yet this mother-daughter conversation illustrates one of the realities of a woman's life. From a very early age women have two primal fears about their breasts: Will they ever grow? Will someone take them away?

Whether we like it or not, admit it or not, our breasts are very much part of our identities. Five-year-old girls begin to anticipate the day when they too will have breasts. Their desire for large breasts—the bigger the better—does not come from five-year-old boys, but from within themselves, from their peers, and from a culture that tells them that bigger is better. Bigger is more powerful, an expression of superiority.

Thirty years later, a woman has come to terms with the size of her breasts and begins to worry about their health. Intensive educational efforts over the last five to ten years have convinced women that the best way to beat breast cancer is to catch it in its earliest stages—even before a lump appears. This is best done with a baseline mammogram, an x-ray of the breast that provides the first map of the area, a map against which future abnormalities or changes can be checked and examined. Conversation among women of a certain age more and more reflects a new orientation—while the fear remains as intense as ever, it is now accompanied by an aggressive need to find cancer before it makes itself too readily apparent.

This is in sharp contrast to the attitudes of women who suffered mutilating surgery and severe psychological trauma only to retreat into the dark shadows of their minds and/or their lives to hide from husbands and loved ones in shame and self-loathing. There are still women who feel shame at the loss of one or both breasts, but the majority now understand that the shame must be dealt with, not hidden or buried. They seek professional counseling or work with volunteers whose own personal experiences have taught them that you are not less of a person—less of a woman—because you are less well endowed.

Despite all this education and enlightened thinking, most women still harbor two distinct and very real fears: (1) that they may have breast cancer, and (2) that their treatment will involve the loss of one or both breasts.

There are not many women alive who can admit to not having these fears. With good reason. Although breast cancer can be an easy cancer to treat medically, it affects one of the few parts of the body that specifically relates to a woman's femininity and feelings of self-worth. Cancer of just about any other part of the body is less of a personal invasion; surgery on any other part of the body—even vaginal surgery—is not likely to be as sensitive a matter.

Breast Facts

As breast-oriented as our culture is, we know very little about the physiology of our breasts. Before we have breasts, all we can wonder is when we'll get them. Once we have breasts, all we can wonder is why they aren't bigger, smaller, rounder, fuller, bouncier, or less bouncy. We've come to know over the years that a lump is a danger signal and that there are "good" lumps and "bad" lumps. Beyond that, most of us are ignorant about the very basics of breasts.

Although both men and women have breasts, women's breasts are more highly evolved because of their role in nurturing the young. Long before there were bottles or formulas, there were breasts. Their role in culture is supposed to be secondary to their role in nature.

The breast is essentially a ball of fatty tissue. It is supported by muscle, but there are no muscles within the breast. Breasts are filled with glands, including the miraculous network that can turn a woman into a milk machine within hours after she has given birth. The shape of the breast can, and does, vary greatly from woman to woman and, every now and then, from breast to breast. (Not everyone has a matched set!)

Doctors believe that both breast cancer and nonmalignant fibrocystic changes begin within the milk ducts and then spread first into the breast tissue and then, if left unchecked, into other parts of the body.

Breast Cancer

Breast cancer is an amazing phenomenon. Although the number of women afflicted has not risen dramatically over the last fifty years, the statistics are changing quickly, because more and more women are summoning the courage to seek treatment before it's too late. Mortalities are stabilized, and although there is a new increase in the number of cases of breast cancer reported among *younger* women (35 to 45 years of age), it is believed that more advanced techniques of diagnosing and treating the disease are responsible for not only the halting death rate but the rising figures of incidence, as well. Since survival is most closely tied to early detection, this is good news for the home team.

With fewer radical mastectomies performed, and more patients considering the option of reconstruction, the number of women willing to take the steps necessary to saving their own lives appears to be increasing. As recently as twenty years ago, a sadly large percentage of women were so embarrassed or so terrified that they preferred to keep their disease a secret—until it was too late. The experience of a new generation of women has proved not only that life is worth living with one breast, but also that medical practices can be changed and improved. Breast cancer and its treatment is an ever-growing, fast-changing field. Advances and improvements are constant—we need only the strength and the courage to cope.

Treatments

The treatment of breast cancer depends on several factors and varies from patient to patient and even from medical team to medical team. For patients who have small tumors and no affected lymph nodes, doctors work to cure the patient and eradicate the disease. For patients whose disease is more involved, there are more involved treatments that may work to cure the patient or simply to keep her alive as long as possible. It is a known fact that without treatment, the breast cancer patient will die, probably within five years.

Treatment of breast cancer will invariably include some type of surgery but may not call for the removal of the affected breast. The days in which a breast and part of the chest wall were immediately removed—in toto—are over. Now, depending on the size of the tumor, adequate but not excessive surgery is performed, followed by radiation and/or chemotherapy.

MASTECTOMY

The *radical mastectomy* was developed at the end of the nineteenth century and was considered the treatment of record until very recently. Grossly lacking in knowledge on the subject, doctors applied the "cut it out" method of saving lives and began performing what is known as the *Halsted* radical mastectomy in 1894, five years after Dr. William S. Halsted had invented the procedure. Halsted believed that the breast, the major and minor pectoral muscles (chest muscles), and the axillary lymph nodes under the arm had to be removed to ensure the patient's life. Few doctors considered the procedure crude or excessive; for more than fifty years it was the undisputed means of treating breast cancer. Women who mourned the loss of their breast were told to be glad they were alive. Indeed, the Halsted was basically the only alternative to death that was offered breast cancer patients until rather recently.

The mutilative effects of the radical mastectomy, coupled with survival data and follow-up statistics that were equally depressing, led to the development of the *modified radical mastectomy*. Here, the axillary nodes are still removed, but the muscles in the chest are not. With the chest muscles left intact, a woman does not suffer the dug-out, hollowed chest that is customary with a radical, but she is still minus one breast. The modified has much of the emotional impact of the Halsted, with the benefit that a perfectly flat chest remains, rather than a disfigured one. This surgery is more complicated than the Halsted but increases the likelihood that the patient may be able to choose reconstruction at a later date.

Unless the cancer is in an advanced stage and may have penetrated the chest wall muscles, most surgeons will now perform this modified radical mastectomy rather than the Halsted. Today the modified is most often called a *total mastectomy with axillary dissection*.

A *simple mastectomy* removes the breast and rarely anything more. It is most commonly used for patients with early breast cancer and is usually followed by radiation treatment. Breast reconstruction can easily be performed at a later date, if desired.

When a tumor is small, and not near the nipple, doctors may suggest a partial mastectomy. This surgery, in which basically just the tumor and the surrounding tissue are taken out, has two forms—the *lumpectomy,* in which just the lump and the tissue immediately surrounding it are removed, and the *segmentectomy,* which usually involves the removal of one-fourth (a quadrant) of the breast—including the lump and more tissue than is removed in the lumpectomy. Both are followed by radiotherapy. Survival rates are excellent.

SAVING THE BREAST

Several states have recently passed laws that require a doctor to tell his patient of the alternatives to the total, or modified radical, mastectomy. Although 80 percent of the patients still choose the simple mastectomy, others are opting to have only the tumor and the immediate area excised, while leaving most of the breast intact. Indeed, so many women have expressed anger at what they consider an unnecessary loss, that clinical research is focusing increasingly on the partial mastectomy alternatives of lumpectomy and segmentectomy.

After a patient has recovered from partial mastectomy surgery and follow-up radiation treatment, the missing section of her breast can be augmented with an implant. Sometimes the breast has healed so nicely that the difference is only slightly noticeable—depending, of course, on the size and shape of the breasts before surgery—in which case no implant may be needed. Since most breast tumors appear in the upper, outer quadrant of the breast, the cosmetic results are usually excellent.

Patient reaction is mixed, as is medical opinion. Many patients are thrilled to have had the more minimal surgery and to keep their breasts. Others feel that there is always room for doubt with the lumpectomy or segmentectomy and fear that because early stages of cancer may have gone undetected in other parts of the breast, they may indeed have a recurrence much sooner than otherwise anticipated. A simple mastectomy is the insurance these patients need in order to believe that they are safe and have done everything they can to prevent further problems.

After a recent ten-year study in Milan, a doctor concluded that, with small tumors, a quadrantectomy accompanied by radiation therapy is equal to a mastectomy in postmenopausal women, in terms of survival statistics and cure rate.

In another larger study, done in the United States, patients who received lumpectomies, with or without radiation, fared "no worse" than the patients who received mastectomies. Dr. Bernard Fisher, of the University of Pittsburgh, led the study but advises that the lumpectomy is not appropriate for all cases of early breast cancer and should not replace the mastectomy. His investigation, he stresses, included only women with tumors less than $1\frac{1}{2}$ inches in diameter and excluded those involving skin or located behind the nipple.

Within the next ten years, a more definitive opinion will be formed on the lumpectomy and each woman will have more choices regarding the surgery that is most appropriate for her—mentally and physically.

RADIATION IMPLANTS

Although radiation treatment for breast cancer patients is not new—it has been used since the mid-1920s—radiation implants have only been around for a few years; but their use in the treatment of certain locally oriented types of cancer is rapidly increasing. One of the doctors pioneering radiation implants is Dr. Samuel Hellman at the Joint Center for Radiation Therapy in Boston, who works most often with lumpectomy patients. After the patient has recovered from surgery, Hellman implants several tiny radiation tubes in her breast, for constant and direct treatment. He later removes the rods, and the implantation site heals with small, circular scars.

Traditional radiation treatment requires x-rays to burn through the skin in order to deliver their deadly dose to the cancer cells beneath. Implants are laid *beneath* the skin and so do less damage to the body— radiation burns are eliminated, as are some of the other side effects of radiation treatment, such as fatigue and lowered white blood count.

Radiation implants work like this: Several (usually eight to twelve) hollow steel needles are inserted into the breast in the quadrant from which the tumor has already been removed. Plastic tubes, or rods, are placed over the needles; then the needles are removed. The remaining tubes are filled with radioactive ingredients that do their work for several days before they are removed. The procedure is done in a hospital and is often called a "booster"—the idea being that the implant teams up with the lumpectomy to eradicate the cancer cells in your breast.

Once removed, implants are not reinserted. If the scars from implants bother you six months after they have completely healed, talk to your dermatologist about the possibility of collagen supplements to fill out the breast and the scars, or you may want to augment the breast through reconstructive surgery.

Radiation implant work is very controversial: it has had mixed results cosmetically and has left many doctors skeptical. It is not uncommon to find a doctor who suggests a simple mastectomy rather than this procedure. Cosmetic success is largely dependent on the original size of the patient's breast and the size of the tumor that has been removed. There may be some shrinkage and discoloration due to radiotherapy. Explore all aspects of this technique before you go for it—especially if your reason for choosing it is cosmetic.

OTHER TREATMENTS

Treatment for breast cancer varies tremendously with the stage of the disease and the patient. A few women just have surgery. Others have surgery accompanied by radiation or radiation implants. (Implants may be coordinated with radiation treatment.) Some women have surgery, radiotherapy, and chemotherapy. If chemotherapy is given, the drugs or combination of drugs chosen will depend on the patient and the medical team. Some breast cancer patients may be candidates for a well-tolerated treatment known as *endocrine therapy*. Usage of this treatment depends on the biologic nature of the individual patient's tumor.

Side effects of treatment will also be individual. At the time of your first consultation with your oncological team, ask about possible side effects with the understanding that some side effects (like hair loss) are expected for a large percentage of patients, whereas others (fatigue, nail damage, skin changes) seem to occur on a per-case basis. There just may be something in your body, unbeknownst to you or your medical team, that will give you the ability to tolerate chemotherapy in a way other patients cannot.

Regardless of the side effects, chemotherapy and radiotherapy are temporary. They will pass.

Recovery

Following breast surgery, you will probably be visited by a volunteer from Reach for Recovery, or another organization that is dedicated to helping mastectomy patients. This volunteer will have had a mastectomy and lived with it for at least one year before qualifying to be in the program that sends her to your bedside. She is, above all, proof that you too can return to a normal lifestyle in a short period of time.

This volunteer will give you brochures, general tips, possibly a rubber ball to exercise with, and as much attention and care as you show her you need. She will also offer her own personal tips. Below are my tips, which are basically for patients who have had radical mastectomies. Patients who have had less extreme surgery will have less difficulty with recovery, at least physically.

- Give yourself time to grieve, hopefully in private or with those closest to you. You cannot be expected to sit in a hospital bed and grin, acting like everything's just fine, thank you. See friends as soon as you are able and have answers to their questions of concern prepared. But don't feel pressured to act as if nothing's wrong. If you don't feel ready to face friends yet, give yourself a little time. If you find that you are hiding, *get some professional help.*

- If you feel you have no one who can understand your current situation, ask for a volunteer, a nurse, or a psychologist to talk to. There are now psychologists who specialize in this area (women who have had mastectomies). Emotional recovery is as important as physical recovery. Many women are afraid to talk to their husbands, lovers, or children about their feelings and intentionally close off these channels of communication. Medical statistics show that men cope much better than women think they will and that women need the reassurance of an understanding mate. Start talking as soon as you are able, and unburden yourself—you will not survive mentally if you lock yourself into self-imposed silence.

- Begin to exercise immediately, even if it's just to squeeze the ball that the volunteer has brought you. (If no free ball is forthcoming, ask a friend or family member to bring you a small rubber ball or even a tennis ball. Keep this at your bedside and squeeze it with your surgical arm when you are watching TV or visiting with friends.) This will help you physically and mentally. You don't have to get compulsive, just get to work. Use the surgical side a little more each day. Continue to exercise after you get home; build up to using weights, slowly but surely. Get maximum use from your surgical side.

- Ask when you can get out of your hospital gown. Some hospitals allow patients to wear their own garments, others do not. All hospitals allow patients to wear their own bathrobes. Bring a nice robe or kimono to the hospital—preferably a big robe or something soft and feminine. Kimonos are particularly nice because they have slits under the armholes to give maximum mobility and drape, are not very expensive (unless you go in for the antique ones), and are beautiful to look at. While you have dressings, you'll want the style of nightgown that opens in the front—even a snap-front coat or dressing gown—rather than a gown that goes over the head.

- Some women like the support and the feeling of a cotton nightgown. A men's undershirt can easily be cut open in front and then safety-pinned—one patient I met asked her daughter to sew Velcro tabs on a few such T-shirts, so that she could open them easily when the doctor came to check her dressings, and then close the shirt snugly for support and comfort.

- For at-home wear immediately following surgery, choose front-buttoning clothes. Anything that has to go over your head will be a bit uncomfortable for a while.

- You should not get a prosthesis until you are healed from surgery and your doctor has given his permission; in the meantime, you may want to place a sock or a wad of cotton in your brassiere to fill out your clothes. Some women feel tremendous pressure to wear a brassiere while in the hospital and to put forward two breasts for their guests. More and more women, however, are accepting of the surgery and never bother with a form or a pretense—while in the hospital or later on. This is a changing style. Do what feels right to you and don't worry about anyone else.

- Once home, pamper your sore side until it heals. Avoid any constriction on this side of your body; don't even wear tight jewelry. Don't let brassiere straps cut into your shoulder or back; wear your handbag on the shoulder that is not affected; carry packages on your good side, not your surgical side. The idea isn't to feel sorry for yourself but to be aware of any circumstance that could lead to a further complication—like infection.

- Wear rubber gloves; garden gloves. Avoid dishpan hands, bruises, cuts, bug bites, cat scratches, or any minor injury that could open up.

- Avoid injections and vaccinations in the arm on your surgery side. Never accept any medical treatment without advising the doctor that you are a cancer patient; always check with your oncologist before accepting medical (or dental) treatment for any condition.

- Discuss all medication with your oncologist—especially hormone-related drugs such as birth control pills for premenopausal women or hormones for postmenopausal women.

- Use a thimble when sewing.

- Use pot holders when cooking; avoid burns with a new resolve. Reach into the oven for dishes with your nonsurgical arm even if this means bringing the pan closer to the mouth of the oven and then using both hands to retrieve the pan. Do not attempt to lift a heavy dish from the oven with only one hand! If you are right-handed and your surgery is on your right side, reach in with the left hand, bring the dish forward, and then use both hands to carry it to the counter.

- Do not use deodorant on your surgical side until you are totally healed from surgery. Switch from brands with aluminum chloride in them—these are usually called "antiperspirants." A regular deodorant will work; if you have a problem, apply again later in the day. While you are recovering, a daily sponge bath will keep odor in check. Use a roll-on deodorant rather than a spray, as the chemicals from the spray can get into the wound and cause irritation. Why ask for trouble?

- Use SPF 15 sunscreen; talk to your doctor about the advisability of sunbathing at all. If you are out in bright sunlight for more than fifteen minutes, make sure your skin is protected against burning. Even if you are not going to have chemotherapy, you should protect your skin against sunburn; there is some concern that sun blocks with a high mineral-oil content may cause skin cancer. Read the label and choose carefully.

- Your driving days may be limited in the beginning, especially if you have bilateral surgery. When friends come to the hospital and ask what they can do for you, sign them up for driving errands or for getting you out of the house. Leave the driving to them. Get car pools and errands organized from your hospital bed—it will give you something to do and will be most helpful in dealing with the frustration that comes when you can't drive.

- Take time for yourself. The best survivors are the happiest survivors—give yourself time to adjust to your new circumstances and then give yourself time to enjoy life. Try to eliminate as much outside stress from your life as possible. If you were superwoman or supermom, play sick for a few months. Don't do as much and you'll live to be a happier person.

The New You

Each woman adjusts to her surgery in her own way, at her own time. Many feel that the loss of a breast is the most terrible thing that can happen to them. Others consider the time spent without a breast as merely a waiting period until they can have reconstruction. A large number of women get along just fine without their breast. "Symmetry," one woman confided to me, "is not what it's cracked up to be."

Your own sense of self is very much related to your body image. Your feelings about yourself and your femininity go back to your childhood and your relationship with your parents. You cannot expect yourself to change overnight or to shrug and say, "I'm just happy to be alive." Of course you are happy to be alive, but if you are to be alive happily, you must come to terms with your new body image. This is an individual matter. I cannot help you here. But I can suggest that every woman deserves some professional help in this area. Don't be shy. If you have been treated in a breast center or a cancer clinic, there's a good chance that there is a staff psychologist on hand to help you. There may be no fee; the fee may be part of your medical package. There are also many support groups and hundreds of thousands of women out there who have had the surgery and who will talk to you, woman to woman. While not every woman will have the same reaction to the surgery, there are those who understand what you are going through and who will help you come to terms with the new you. Don't deny them, or yourself.

You will never be well until you heal the emotional scars.

Breast Tricks

Whether you've had one or both breasts removed, there are several tricks that you can perform in the privacy of your home that will convince the public that your figure is everything it should be.

Depending on the original size of your breasts, you will decide if you want a breast prosthesis and what kind. Women with small- to average-size breasts often decide to go braless (and prosthesisless), to use a lightly molded or padded bra and no prosthesis, or to use a homemade prosthesis and forget about anything more fancy. Women with larger breasts often have a balance problem without a prosthesis—they may even need weighted prosthetic devices. Because a large breast can easily weigh five pounds, a mastectomy may produce an immediate weight loss and cause unusual strain on the back. Large-breasted women, especially, need to have expert advice in the fitting of prosthetic devices and on the right way to sit, rise, and walk during the time before a weighted prosthesis can be used.

Although most doctors advise their patients to wait before purchasing a more permanent prosthesis, even those patients who are planning on reconstruction usually augment their breast in some way. (Some patients have a lumpectomy first and then a prophylactic mastectomy with implants. See Reconstruction below.) You can use light cotton padding in your regular brassiere while you are in the hospital and during the healing period after. You may also want to use a polyester form (you may be given one by a volunteer or purchase one in the hospital) or even a sock. Don't laugh—socks are very popular with breast cancer patients. Since many doctors like reconstruction patients to wait one year before they are "rebuilt," many a woman has left the hospital wearing three socks and laughing wryly.

There are two types of commercial prosthetics for breast cancer patients—and many brands within the types. For patients who have had a Halsted or even a modified radical, there is a breast form that is shaped like a comma—the extra piece helps fill out the chest wall or the hollow area under the arm or under the collarbone. Then there are the plain old regular prosthetic breast forms, which now come in many different textures—without deviating too dramatically from its intended purpose of being a breast form. This is a growing area of concern, and more and more types of forms are becoming available. Choose from breasts that can actually be taped directly to the body or forms that are made of gels and feel exactly like a real breast. Stay tuned and ask around before you make a decision in this department. Use some of your recovery time at home to make phone calls; find out what's available in your area and in the largest city near you.

A commercial prosthesis is by no means a woman's only choice. There are the obvious homemade devices—like wads of cotton, or socks—and the more sophisticated devices that just take a little bit of craftiness. Breast pads have long been sold in stores, for insertion in bathing suits and brassieres. My favorite breast form trick was learned behind closed closet doors at the studio of designer Bob Mackie. I call it, simply enough, the Bob Mackie trick, and mastectomy patients have had stunning results with it.

The weight of a beaded dress (from 20 to 50 pounds!) can make even a large-breasted woman look flat-chested. To offset this problem, Mackie sews a set of breast forms into many of the gowns he makes. If you're familiar with Mackie's more spectacular creations, you know that many of them have no back, no sides, and very little front. How does he get the pads in, and what are they attached to so that you can't see them? I thought you'd never ask.

Mackie covers regular old breast pads (bought at a home sewing store) with fabric that matches the dress or with nude-colored soufflé—a fabric that is a lot like chiffon. The form is covered with two matching ovals of cloth that are larger than the breast form and are attached by tiny hand stitches around the edges of the form. Excess fabric is then trimmed away, leaving just enough to tack the now-covered breast form into the front of the dress. You now have an instant strapless, backless, and sideless brassiere. For the mastectomy patient who wishes to wear a strapless, backless, or partially frontless dress or evening gown, this method is sensational. (If chiffon itches, try cutting up an old pair of pantyhose.) Various less dramatic techniques can be applied with breast pads, homemade pockets in existing brassieres, and store-bought padded brassieres.

If you have a homemade breast form, don't forget about the Betty Rollin trick, which is almost as good as the Bob Mackie trick. Sew a button to your form, or inside the cup of your brassiere—this will protrude just as your nipple does if you are one of those women who wear a natural-style brassiere. Experiment with different buttons until you get the exact size, shape, and degree of protrusion that you want. You can judge only when you are wearing a T-shirt, so be prepared for a bit of trying on and fooling around.

Buying a Breast

As recently as fifteen years ago, information about breast prostheses was passed from woman to woman as a secret that only those who needed to know knew. There were no specialty shops in those days, and the postmastectomy patient was sent to the lingerie department of a big department store where she was to whisper her mission as if she was a spy in a Robert Ludlum novel. "I'd like to see someone about a breast prosthesis," she would say with all the dignity she could muster.

The saleswoman would turn pale and say, "Oh, you want Mrs. So and So."

It was awkward, painful, embarrassing, and demeaning.

Now, most of the prosthesis business has moved out of the department stores. Hospitals and medical supply houses continue to sell the items, but specialty stores now get the most business. If there isn't one in your community, perhaps you can visit a nearby large city.

Even women who are happy with their homemade prosthetic devices like to know what's on the market; sometimes they even shop around. Some buy several styles over a period of time. Others find a store-bought prosthesis a silly waste (a fancier one can cost $250 to $500) and are happy with the money they have saved.

One woman may go to a shop that specializes in clothing and intimate apparel for breast cancer patients, expecting to find someone knowledgable and sympathetic, and end up in tears of hurt and shock. Another woman may go to a similar shop and find she is treated with open arms, lots of warmth, and caring comments about her scar or healing process.

"They were real nice to me," says one patient. "It was like a sorority house or something. All the women got together and showed their scars and tried on different forms. I think there's a lot of therapy involved in talking about it and dealing with it among other women who know what you're talking about. This is the kind of thing that your best friend can't help you with unless your best friend has also had a mastectomy."

"I was not at all prepared for it," says a woman who had a contradictory experience. "I thought I'd go to this little shop that the hospital told me about and I would learn everything there. Instead I was bombarded with decisions to make and a lot of pressure and not one bit of understanding."

It's important for you to know that no matter where you go, the search for a bought breast can be a traumatic experience. Take a friend with you. There are few people who should go on this adventure alone, especially the first time out. Most should plan on making an occasion of it: a look-see at a specialty shop, followed by a nice lunch and maybe a somewhat extravagant—and feminine—purchase.

"I tell all my patients to take their best friend with them, then go for the fanciest lunch they can afford, and then go on a shopping spree to a store they can barely afford and buy themselves a soft, feminine blouse that will always make them feel divine," says one nurse.

If you are seriously shopping for a prosthesis, call and make an appointment with the right shop in your area. Go to more than one shop if you can; compare the information you receive. Do not go on this outing if you are feeling tired or upset. Allow at least half an hour for your questions and fitting. Don't rush through it. You are not buying the ingredients for a cake.

Do not be pressured by the sales help. If you feel they are making too strong a pitch or that you are getting upset, leave. Don't stay around to be a nice person. Specialty shops provide a very specific service—

you have a need and they have the knowledge. If the sales help cannot give you the information you desire and let you make your own choice, show them that you are unhappy. Gain as much information as you can before you choose, and make it clear that you wish to make an informed decision. You do not need to buy the first time or at the first place you go shopping.

Salespeople know that this is a vulnerable time in your life. Some will try to mother you, some will treat you as if you don't know what's best for yourself. Others will be helpful and supportive; but do not go on a breast-buying adventure without a good sense of yourself and your needs. Make a list of your questions, or ask some of these:

- I've heard so much about the different types of breast forms. Can you explain them all to me?

- How is it worn/attached? Will you show me?

- Does it take some getting used to? Will I get a rash or irritation at first? Should I build up time using it slowly?

- Can I go swimming with it?

- Can I sleep in it if I want to?

- If it doesn't have a nipple, will the nipple on my other breast show through?

- Will it ride up during the day?

- If someone touches me, or just bumps into me, will he know my secret?

- How do I care for it? Can I wash it? How long does it take to dry? Should I own several? What about traveling? Do I wash it out with Woolite as I do my clothes?

- Will it leak on airplanes?

- Do the tape-on ones really stay on?

- How much does it cost, and how often will it need to be replaced?

- Do I need the request for a prosthesis written on a prescription pad from my doctor so that my insurance will cover this expense?

Breast protheses vary in price tremendously—there are breast forms for $5 and some for $500. The average price is well under $100, and most health insurance plans pay for the device. The price range varies so greatly because of the many types of devices available and their varying composition. Prostheses, just like other products, are available in designer styles. Some brands advertise famous personalities and may be more costly as a result.

Don't forget to ask your doctor to write you a prescription for a breast prosthesis—this will make it tax-deductible, in the event that your health insurance doesn't pay for all of this expense. (Your wig should also be written on a prescription pad as a medical prosthetic device.)

Reconstruction

As women have communicated feelings of mutilation and betrayal that accompanied their mastectomies, advances in medical research have been aimed toward helping them adjust to the loss of the breast—or preventing the spread of cancer while actually saving the breast. The most exciting strides have been made in the field of breast reconstruction, a more or less new procedure. While the new breast will never be identical to the one that was forfeited to surgery, it is indeed a breast. Beyond that, it bounces, sags, looks, and feels like a breast and in a few cases is even *better* than the one that Mother Nature provided.

It is not unusual for a reconstruction patient to have work done on both sides of her chest—a new breast is built by a plastic surgeon and then the existing breast is modified (augmented or reduced), to provide the owner with what's commonly referred to as "a very nice set."

An even newer type of reconstruction is emerging in which the patient never loses her own breasts. The tumor is removed by means of a lumpectomy. The patient heals, has radiotherapy and/or chemotherapy, and *then* returns for one operation in which her own breast is removed and a new one built, or her own breast tissue is removed and implants are inserted beneath her skin. This way the patient never goes through any period of time without a breast. This method is particularly popular among bilateral patients and women who have a high chance of a recurrence in the second breast.

Reconstruction methods continue to change and improve. Talk to your doctors and several plastic surgeons about the possibilities before you decide which type of surgery to have. If a new method is being perfected, investigate it and the surgeons who have had the most practice applying it—you may want to consider flying to a different city for your surgery.

Approximately 80 percent of the women who have mastectomies are candidates for reconsuction, and this figure is rising each day. In the past, few took advantage of the opportunity; but as methods become better known and more successful, more and more women are choosing this option. The most important thing a reconstruction patient should remembr is that the surgery is meant to correct a figure problem *with clothes on.* A rebuilt or new breast may not look like the old one and may not qualify the owner for a title at the next Ms. Nude America pageant. There have been stories of botched jobs and women who were sorry they had the surgery. On the other hand, reconstruction does put something in the brassiere and fills out the lines of a garment. It provides cleavage and bounce and eliminates the self-conscious worry of "will they know I'm wearing a prosthesis?" The new surgery is considered no less than a miracle by thousands of women who have undergone it.

"I never went through the loss of my breasts, so I didn't have any stigma or trauma to deal with. The doctors figured I had had cancer for five to seven years before it was discovered, and that put me at a high risk for a recurrence. When I found out about bilateral surgery, I decided to have both done at the same time. After the chemo, I went back for the implants. The doctor said he squeezed a size-ten foot into a size-six shoe. He certainly gave me more than what I started out with. I kept asking for bigger. But I'm real satisfied with them. I don't wear a brassiere, they don't sag. I think it's a miracle. If it helps anyone else to know about it, they can call me. I feel very confident about my future and I have no complaints about breast surgery. The chemo was very hard on me, but the rest has been very exciting."

Women over 65 rarely choose reconstruction—not because they are afraid, uninterested in the idea, or happy the way they are, but because they aren't interested in undergoing additional surgery. Most say they wish they had had an opportunity when they were younger, that such surgery could have made them feel a lot better about themselves and their bodies. The younger the patient, the more inclined she is toward reconstruction.

Reconstructive surgery is not necessarily that difficult. For a woman who's had a modified radical mastectomy, in which the chest muscles are left intact, the procedure is straightforward—a plastic surgeon opens up the chest wall under local or general anesthetic, creates a pocket between the skin and the muscles, and inserts an implant—the kind that models, movie stars, and Hollywood wives are known to favor. The surgery is considered very safe, essentially risk-free. A nipple is usually created later, in a second operation. During either the first or the second surgery, the unaffected breast may also be operated on, to adjust it to the size and shape of the new breast. Small-breasted women can augment their remaining natural breast with an implant to make it the same size as the new breast. Women with larger breasts can have a big bosom reduced in size. The patient is often in and out of the hospital in twenty-four to thirty-six hours.

The operation is more complicated if the chest muscle has to be replaced, or if there isn't enough skin available to create the new breast. In these cases, doctors take a donation from another part of the patient's body—usually the back—and create the breast from a football-shaped flap of skin. Muscle, too, can be taken from the back. This surgery is naturally more involved and requires approximately a two-week hospital stay. Another technique, not as popular, takes the flap of skin from the abdomen so that the patient gets a free tummy tuck in the process. This is still considered controversial, so investigate all other methods before signing up for it.

There is some scarring with reconstruction, depending on the type of surgery and how well an individual's body heals. The scars are usually in the lower half of the breast and on other private parts.

The cost of reconstruction varies with the surgeon and the city in which he operates, as well as with the difficulty of the task. Simple work begins at $2500; more complicated reconstruction costs $5000 to $6000. Reconstructive surgery is considered safe and there are few problems associated with it. The most common problem is a hardening of the tissue around the implants. Some reconstruction patients have to have surgery to replace their implants every two to three years. This takes time and money, but health insurance should cover much of the cost.

Immediate Gratification

Whether you are a candidate for immediate reconstruction depends mostly on how large your tumor is and what complete treatment your medical team advises. For people with a more advanced stage of cancer, a larger tumor, and possible lymph node involvement, doctors often suggest an immediate mastectomy, followed by a program of radiotherapy and chemotherapy, and then reconstruction six to twelve months after the end of treatment. This gives the patient time to regain her health and come to grips with the trauma created by the sudden discovery of a tumor. This also gives the skin time to regain its elasticity.

Because it is not uncommon for a woman to delay seeking medical advice once she discovers a lump, for fear that loss of her breast is imminent, the knowledge that immediate reconstruction is possible is a tremendous boon to the shy and the terrified. Early detection is by far the best means of achieving victory over cancer—perhaps the knowledge that breasts can be saved and/or immediately rebuilt will bring more and more women into treatment.

Doctors do warn that patients who choose immediate reconstruction must have realistic expectations of their new breast. Since these women have not already been through the trauma of having no breast at all, they are not as likely to appreciate what the surgeon can and cannot do. Just as a wig is not the same as your lost hair, a reconstructed breast will never be the same as a biological breast. Failure to understand this point and to think through the situation seriously can lead to hurt, disappointment, and serious psychological trauma. The woman who has lived without one or both breasts is happy for whatever improvements the doctor can make; the woman who has never come to terms with her illness may find herself unprepared emotionally for the true meaning of "immediate reconstruction."

Again, even with immediate reconstruction, a second operation is needed later—for placement of the new nipple and possible adjustments in symmetry and size.

The Waiting Game

Knowledge that reconstruction is available is the carrot on the stick that satisfies many breast cancer patients. The period between mastectomy and reconstruction can be a valuable time for them personally—they have come to terms with themselves and their bodies, and with their role as women at home and in society. The time may have been painful, but they usually admit they have grown from the experience.

Patients who choose to wait before undertaking reconstruction usually wait a year and then begin to interview plastic surgeons and investigate the right steps for them. One of the great things about reconstruction is that in most cases it can be done after any length of time—one year, ten years, or more. It's not unusual for a woman to change her lifestyle and then want reconstruction.

Furthermore, reconstruction is becoming increasingly advanced as each year passes. It's still a developing art. Most doctors now feel they do better work on a postmastectomy basis, but as techniques are improved, immediate breast removal and reconstruction will become more and more common.

Nipples

Nipples are created from grafted skin and are usually attached to a reconstructed breast in a second operation. Some women choose not to have a nipple attached. Doctors don't ordinarily save the patient's original nipple, because of the finer network of blood vessels and glands that could well host invisible but nonetheless lethal cancer cells. However, with small tumors that were not located near the nipple, surgeons may indeed favor a process called *nipple banking.* At the time of the mastectomy, the patient's nipple is "banked," or saved in another part of the body—often the labia—until it can be retrieved for reconstruction. Before a nipple can be banked, it must be sent to the pathologist for a thorough checkup to ensure that no cancer is present. Yet the possibility of invisible cancer is so frightening to some doctors that they do not advocate nipple banking.

There are a few methods for creating new nipples. Some surgeons remove the one remaining, safe nipple, cut it in half, and rebuild it into two smaller, matching nipples. Other surgeons prefer to graft skin from the labia or from behind the ear to create a new nipple.

For women with large or spread nipples, surgery to reduce the nipple's size (on the unaffected breast) is often performed to match the nipples in size if not in actual shape. Nipple grafting or reconstruction is usually done several months after actual breast reconstruction, so that the new breast has a chance to settle.

Preventive Mastectomy

As implants and immediate reconstructive surgery techniques are perfected, a growing number of women are considering *preventive mastectomies*—surgery performed *before* there is evidence of cancer. These women are invariably high-risk candidates, including patients who have had one mastectomy and been advised that there is a strong likelihood that they will in time develop cancer in the second breast as well.

Preventive, also called *prophylactic*, mastectomy is considered extremely controversial, especially for women with totally healthy breasts. For high-risk women who have already had one mastectomy, bilateral surgery as a preventive method of treatment is not uncommon.

Women who have had a preventive mastectomy use advanced methods of mammography (xeroxography or thermography) to keep track of the health of their breasts. Preventive mastectomy does not preclude the possibility of a recurrence or of new cancer developing somewhere else at a future date, so self-examination and mammography procedures must be strictly followed.

Ostomies

An *ostomy* is a surgical procedure by which a plug is inserted into the abdomen for the control of personal waste matter. It is necessitated by certain types of cancer that destroy the parts of the body that provide for the regular elimination process. The actual opening created is called a *stoma*.

There are currently over one million ostomates (or people with ostomies) living in the United States and Canada, so you are not alone with this problem. There is no reason to be afraid or embarrassed. There is every reason to learn as much as you can so that you can have the independence you crave.

Ostomy surgery is performed for several different types of cancer, including bladder and bowel cancer. However, an ostomy is not performed on every patient who has one of these forms of cancer.

- The *descending,* or *sigmoid, colostomy* is performed when the left colon or the rectum is diseased, damaged, or removed.

- The *transverse* colostomy is required when the lower stool is blocked or removed. It may be either a temporary or a permanent measure.

- The *urostomy* is a urinary diversion that is required when the bladder or the ureter is damaged or removed.

- The *ileostomy* is performed when the whole colon is damaged, diseased, or removed.

There is a basic emotional turmoil that often accompanies this type of surgery, regardless of the patient's age and sex, or of the type of ostomy performed. However, the patient's ability to deal with her illness is the key to overcoming fears about the need for an ostomy. Education and experience are all it takes for an ostomate to lead a relatively normal life.

As an ostomy patient, you have three major concerns:

1. You want to know that the surgery was worth it—that you will live and be able to cope with the ostomy and not be so embarrassed that your life is ruined.

2. You want to know that you will be independent—that you will be able to care for the device yourself, be able to come and go as you please and not be limited to the places where you may go.

3. You need to rebuild your own body image so that every day becomes a more positive experience; after your discharge from the hospital, you have a lot of mental homework to do.

Luckily, once you understand how your ostomy works and that improvements are made constantly, you will gain confidence and feel less embarrassed and less homebound. Ostomy patients are ones who are afraid—not only are they afraid that they will die (as all cancer patients are) but they are afraid of society's reaction to their problem—they worry about rejection. They are often ashamed, wishing they could have a more public type of cancer that people would understand a little better. They are afraid they can't have sex. They can! They are afraid that they are freaks. They're not!

"I just tell people when they walk in the door and sit down at my house that I have no control over my functions and that anything can happen at any time," says one woman who is learning to live with her situation. "I guess I shouldn't even mention it, or should try to act as if everything is normal, but people aren't coming over to visit because everything's normal in the first place. I guess that fair warning is fair play. If I gurgle or pass wind, I don't want to feel any worse than I already do. There's just nothing worse than being as old as I am and feeling like a damned kid and being so embarrassed that I almost want to cry. So I just play it the other way and make all my announcements up front. Maybe that's not very subtle, but it works for me."

Not all ostomates need worry about "bulges," odors, and noises. A "continent ostomy" is performed on some patients, allowing them to insert the ostomy appliance within a flap of skin. This surgery (which not everyone qualifies for) is the most cosmetically satisfying of any ostomy; yet patients with out-of-the-body appliances, too, can have as flat a tummy as they had before, and can wear bathing suits without anyone knowing their secret. Odors depend on the location of the ostomy but are taken care of by deodorants that are applied to the pouches. Diet control also helps odor control. While gas does make noise, it doesn't happen very often and sounds more like a gurgle than a whoopee cushion. Again, diet control can help control gas.

Caring for an Ostomy

You will be taught to care for your ostomy first by watching your nurse while you are in the hospital, then by her active lessons, and finally by doing it yourself. Some people learn quickly, others fight the idea of learning self-care. This is an individual matter related to the patient's state of readiness for change.

There are different types of equipment and appliances for different types of surgery, different levels of convenience, and different budgets. (Your health insurance should cover most of your expenses.) Ask to see everything and have the differences in the equipment explained to you. Practice and see what feels right to you. Seek the aid of an enterstomal therapist or nurse—it's her job to know what's available and to help you adjust. There are clubs for ostomates; the Ostomal Society publishes a newsletter; there is even an annual ostomate convention.

"I don't need to tell you that I didn't like the idea of an ostomy, but I said 'OK, this is it, it's better than being dead,' and I went on with my life. I never could quite get the hang of the whole thing, but I just figured that was that and I wasn't going to complain. Sometimes I would get frustrated and be near tears, but I never complained to anyone. I went in to my doctor for a checkup one day, and the nurse showed me this type of equipment that had been available all along; it was like night and day. I got everything changed around and my life is so much better, I can't tell you. I don't know whose fault it was that I didn't find out about everything the first time around, but it pays to ask a lot of questions and be nosy. Don't suffer because you think you are supposed to."

Gynecologic Matters

"Plumbing"

Twenty years ago, when a woman had gynecologic surgery, she smiled mysteriously and said she was having her "plumbing" fixed. This usually meant she was having a hysterectomy, but the phrase covered a wide range of possibilities and made it clear that an unspeakable part of her body was being operated on and that no more need be said.

When mum's the word, women suffer. While uterine and ovarian cancer and their treatment are more openly discussed than, say, cancer of the vulva, many women feel uncomfortable talking about these problems or admitting to having them. No matter what their age, no matter how many children they have, they feel that loss of an ovary or loss of the uterus threatens their sexuality and/or their femininity.

Many women feel that cancer of the private parts is preferable to breast cancer—breast cancer can be obvious from a cosmetic standpoint, whereas gynecologic cancer is not. Other women have a genuine terror of losing what they claim is the true definition of their womanhood—their periods. This is an individual matter, but also appears to be age-related. Premenopausal women are the most upset about the supposed loss of femininity; postmenopausal women have already dealt with their change of life and are therefore not so emotionally attached to their "plumbing."

From the standpoint of sexual pleasure, little is different, explains Dr. Robert Futoran, an oncological gynecologist in Beverly Hills. "For the patient who is having a hysterectomy, nothing will change. For the patient who is having a vulvectomy, I ask if she has internal or external climaxes. If the answer is external, then her sex life will change because the clitoris is removed—otherwise, her sex life can be the same as before."

The incidence of gynecologic cancer in women under the age of 60 is low, and so the cosmetic problems associated with the disease are minimal. Many women who have already stopped having sex do not feel terribly traumatized by gynecologic surgery. But some patients who lose a vagina to surgery will ask to have a new one constructed. The reconstructed vagina will enable the woman to have regular sexual relations but is often requested not for sexual purposes, but for insurance reasons. Some women like to know they have a vagina so that, on subsequent checkups, their doctor can make sure it is cancer-free.

For women who have vaginal radiation implants, there are usually no further cosmetic complications. The implants are done in a hospital, just like breast implants (see Radiation Implants, above) and are removed in the hospital. There is no scarring. Although some patients complain of the cosmetic aftereffects of radiation implants in breasts (possible scars, shrinkage), there are no such complaints about vaginal implants.

Doctors notice that the younger the woman, the more difficulties she has in dealing with gynecologic cancer and her own sexuality. Age seems to be a great begetter of wisdom:

- The 40-year-old patient says: Why me, God?

- The 60-year-old patient says: Thank God I didn't need a colostomy.

- The 70-year-old patient says: Thank God I'm alive.

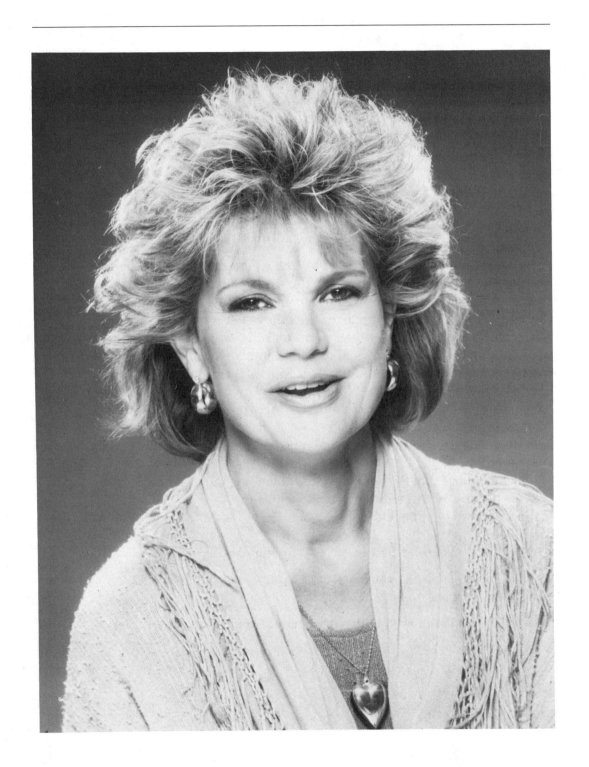

Chapter Seven

DIET AND EXERCISE

Figure Control

During World War I, many women complained that the men left behind were "either too young or too old." Cancer patients have a similar complaint, but it's about their weight: they're either too fat or too thin. Very few are satisfied with their figures while they are undergoing chemotherapy. Understandably so.

"It was the last straw," says one breast cancer patient. "First they took away my breast, then they took away my hair. On top of that, the chemo made me fat—I gained ten pounds!"

"I normally pride myself on my looks," explains a uterine cancer patient, "but all that radiation treatment made me so sick I couldn't look at food. I lost and lost. I got like a scarecrow. I looked awful, just awful. The doctor told me I had to gain weight, but I just couldn't imagine eating anything. It took about two weeks for me to be able to just tolerate looking at food, after the treatments were all over. Now it's been a few months, and I've gained back my weight, so I look fine. It takes time, and patience, and some understanding that this is going to happen to you. Of all the side effects, my doctor didn't tell me anything about this one. It's really hard to convince your friends that you're fine and you're going to make it when you look so sick and so thin."

That old expression "You can never be too rich or too thin" just doesn't apply to chemo patients—you really *can* get too thin. Doctors don't usually worry too much about the patient who gains some weight, but the patient who loses weight is a source of concern. Doctors, of course, are not worried about the cosmetic effects of being too thin. They do worry about your body having the strength and resistance to fight off infection; they want your body to function smoothly without interference from medical techniques.

Among mastectomy patients, however, there is a special problem: weight gain is considered part of the recovery process. A mastectomy patient may gain weight from her chemo, which is an acceptable weight gain and must be tolerated. She may also gain weight because she suffers from the "Why me?" syndrome. Why Me syndrome is a state of depression and anxiety that causes many patients to overeat—they tell themselves that they can splurge just this once, or at this vulnerable time, because they have had such a serious trauma; that they are due a reward; that they are so lucky to be alive they are entitled to indulge a little now to make things better. Some overeat as a "replacement" strategy—they are eating to replace what has been lost to them. People who are emotional eaters in the first place—who equate eating with "making it better" may overindulge following any type of surgery. Some will come to grips with their psychological state and pull themselves together; others will never drop the extra weight, simply because they don't want to.

Chemo-related weight gains are very specific. The patient gains seven to eight pounds, rarely as much as ten. Ask your doctor if your drugs are the type that usually bring a weight gain so that you can be prepared. Do not try to fit into your regular clothes or buy one ugly sack dress and say to yourself, "This is temporary, so why spend money on clothes?" If your clothes are tight, uncomfortable, or ill-fitting, you will be more upset than ever. Since the chemo treatment will possibly last six months to a year, you owe it to yourself to be prepared for this weight gain and to splurge on some new clothes that will make you feel as attractive as possible. Borrow some clothes if you can, or buy a few comfortable but nice new outfits. A ten-pound weight gain will probably put you into the next size of clothing; do yourself— and those who love you—a big favor and spring for the more ample clothes. You bought maternity clothes for a real need, didn't you? This is just as important, if not more so. Get the kind of clothes you love, that make you feel good, that you don't mind wearing all the time.

You'll never regret it. When you're off chemo and have reduced to your normal size, take pleasure in giving the clothes away to someone who needs them. Indulge and make your life better!

During chemo and radiation treatment you certainly should not worry about being overweight—it's not a time for fad diets, reducing diets, big adventures at the gymnasium, or hours of dedication to one's favorite Nautilus machine. Since the average weight gain from chemotherapy is under ten pounds, keep vigil at your scale and follow the tips below. If you gain over ten pounds, discuss it with your doctor. WARNING: **Do not attempt a diet without medical advice.**

- Do not fast without permission from your doctor.

- Do not switch to a liquid diet of any kind without permission from your doctor.

- Do not take diet pills of any kind, with or without a prescription.

- Do not adapt a diet from a best-selling book just because it seems to be working for other people; check with your doctor first.

- Do not get involved in a diet that advises use of artificial products or chemicals to enhance or disguise the taste of food or that creates low-calorie foods with chemicals; these chemicals may be carcinogens.

- Do watch the fat content and caffeine levels of the food you are eating; learn more about the possible connection between diet and cancer.

If you are having trouble eating or feel the need to gain weight, talk to your doctor and to other patients who may be able to give you some tips.

- Investigate liquid-food products—several companies make milk-shake drinks that contain all the basic nutrients you need and can keep you happy and healthy during those periods in which food may not be appealing to you. Some of the brand names are Ensure, Isocal, Isomil, Carnation Instant Breakfast, Sustacal (which also comes in a pudding formula), Citrotein, and Meritene. Do not create a diet for yourself, but consider such foods on days when nothing else will go down.

- If you are receiving radiotherapy and find yourself having trouble swallowing or eating, talk to your doctor or nurse about a special diet. The American Cancer Society and many doctors recommend a diet that reads something like the menu that follows.

BREAKFAST

4 ounces orange juice

1 soft-boiled egg or 4 ounces farina cereal

1 slice enriched white toast with 2 teaspoons butter or margarine and/or jam

1 cup coffee

LUNCH

3 ounces chickenburger

1 small baked potato

4 ounces pureed vegetable

1 soft roll with 2 teaspoons butter or margarine

1 cup tea

DINNER

4 ounces clear or cream soup

3 ounces ground beef

1 mashed potato

4 ounces diced or pureed vegetable

1 slice light rye bread

2 teaspoons butter or margarine

1 scoop vanilla ice cream

SNACK

4 ounces applesauce

This type of diet is by no means for everyone; it's just a sample provided by the American Cancer Society. You may want to lay off the coffee and the orange juice and stick with clear liquids—apple juice, seltzer, soup.

Even if you don't feel hungry, eat something on treatment days. It's much easier for your body if it has something in it to throw up. "Dry heaves" are worse than vomiting.

Mini-Meals

For people who complain that food just doesn't taste good, or that they can't even stand the sight of it, doctors suggest a series of snacks during the day—usually six, spread out from morning until bedtime—that will add nutrients to the body but will not put pressure on the patient to sit down and stare at a lot of food.

If you can't eat three regular meals a day, don't worry—many patients can't. Try six mini-meals instead. Repeat foods that appeal to you. Don't tell yourself you have to eat six different meals. Try to vary the food just enough that you don't become constipated—a problem often made worse by chemotherapy drugs.

Remember that a milk shake with an egg in it counts as a mini-meal. If you ever wanted to live on ice cream, now is the time to do it. There are also ice-cream-like nutritional drinks that make ideal mini-meals.

Mother Was Right

No matter what your reaction to food—love it or hate it—during this time period, it is important to keep your body as healthy as possible. According to the National Cancer Institute, Mother was right: food is the fuel your body needs to run.

- Doctors and researchers find that those patients who continue to eat well during treatment have less discomfort and tolerate the treatments much better than those who lose weight and interest in food.

- By eating well, you are helping your body to fight back. Chemo and radiation destroy some cells—naturally they destroy cancer cells, but they also eliminate healthy cells. Eating well helps your body rebuild its losses at a faster rate. The treatment prevents the cancer cells from replenishing themselves, while the well-balanced meals help the body to build new strong, healthy tissue.

- Doctors have found a direct correlation in cancer patients between good eating habits and a lowered number of infections. Give food a chance.

Food Aversions

Some chemo patients develop food aversions during their treatment. While an aversion can come up virtually overnight, usually the syndrome works something like this:

1. You know that you are going for a chemo treatment tomorrow and that you will be ill; it will not be fun.

2. As a treat, sort of the carrot on the stick, you decide to reward yourself with one of your favorite foods.

3. You eat the food and enjoy it and then go for chemo.

4. The food comes back up shortly after chemo.

5. Your mind associates the discomforts of chemo with the food that has heretofore been a favorite.

6. The next time you see or smell that food, you become violently ill.

Tests done on patients who were given ice cream prior to chemo showed that aversions could be attached to even the most attractive of foods; the patients tested all ended up hating ice cream.

Many food aversions last. Others are temporary; like some women during their first months of pregnancy, patients may lose their taste for certain foods and regain a craving for them later. Most aversions end within a year after cessation of chemo. (Aversions may be to things other than food—some people have the same reaction to the smell of disinfectant or to the color green on a hospital's walls.)

If you suffer from an aversion, try to isolate what caused it. Do not eat your favorite foods *before* chemo! Try to prevent new aversions from developing. You should eat before chemo, but stick to simple foods and/or dry toast. Most people who have trouble eating or gaining satisfaction with taste are happiest with light foods such as eggs, pasta, chicken, milk products, and fresh fruits and vegetables.

Vitamins

Most doctors are not as enthusiastic about vitamin pills as other health, beauty, and laypeople are. There have been specific medical tests on the effects of vitamin therapy on cancer—especially with vitamin C and vitamin E—and some hospitals are treating cancer patients with megadoses of these vitamins.

Talk to your own doctor about the role of vitamins in your treatment. Do not prescribe megadoses of anything for yourself. (This can be hazardous to your health.) If you feel that your personal medical community is ignoring your need for vitamins, do some reading on the subject and seek the advice of specialists. Perhaps one of the medical facilities now doing extensive work with cancer and vitamin therapy is located near you.

Multiple vitamins on a daily basis, taken as prescribed, are usually an acceptable boost to Mother Nature.

Calorie Counting

Whether you need to gain weight or lose weight, it's a good idea to buy yourself a paperback calorie-counting encyclopedia. (Get a used one at a book sale for under $1.) In your spare time, read through the listings to acquaint yourself with the high-calorie foods. If you need to gain weight, incorporate those that are appropriate into your diet. If you need to lose weight, avoid those foods or make substitutions.

For example, mayonnaise is high in calories. If you want to gain weight, use it in your dressing preparations. If you need to lose weight, substitute plain low-fat yogurt and save approximately 100 calories per teaspoon.

No one wants to spend time counting calories or being tied to a scale, but a working knowledge of calorie counts is important for everyone—cancer patient or not. Since fattening foods are high in fats, a suspected agent in the cause of some cancers, follow a low-fat "pro-life" diet. It will help you to keep slim and also might fight a possible future invasion of cancer.

Bloating

A few cancer patients complain of bloating—from either water weight or constipation. Bloating may also cause swelling in the face or puffiness that is considered a cosmetic problem. If you find yourself bloated, discuss the situation with your doctor and try some of these tips:

- Ask your doctor about a diuretic. If you do take a diuretic, make sure you eat properly and drink plenty of water to keep your liquids flushed. Many people think that because they are retaining water, they shouldn't drink more water. This is wrong. Drinking water is still one of the best ways to move your system along. If a diuretic has no water to drain out of your body, it will take nutrients that you desperately need. Get complete instructions on the use of diuretics and follow directions to a T.

- Place a brick carefully under each of the legs at the head of the bed and raise that end by a few inches so that your head is slightly higher than your feet. This will help prevent or reduce swelling in your face.

- Many drugs do cause constipation. Consider dietary changes that will help your bowel movements in a natural way before you resort to drugs or laxatives. Never prescribe a laxative for yourself without consulting your doctor. Do not increase the fiber content in your diet without discussing this technique with your doctor—the lining of your intestines may be too sensitive for excessive roughage.

- While some premenopausal women temporarily lose their periods during chemotherapy, those who do not may find bloating a problem prior to their period. This is not uncommon for women without cancer, but chemo may cause more discomfort than usual. Discuss the problem with a doctor. Do not self-prescribe a diuretic while you are undergoing chemotherapy. Talk to your doctor first.

- Do not give yourself an enema without consulting your doctor first.

- Do not make yourself throw up because you feel bloated and think this might make you feel better.

Soft and Simple

The majority of chemo and radiation patients report that they have the most success, especially on treatment days, with foods that are soft and simple. Many eat breakfast foods three times a day. One patient suggests pancakes—vary the ingredients in the batter slightly for some different tastes: add orange juice instead of water to a commercial mix; use sour cream or *crème fraîche* or plain low-fat yogurt. Try crepes with a variety of fillings.

JUDY'S *CRÈME FRAÎCHE* PANCAKES

> 8 ounces store-bought *crème fraîche* (dairy department or gourmet food store)
>
> 8 ounces sifted flour
>
> 1 egg

Mix egg and *crème fraîche*. Add sifted flour and mix. Drop with soup spoon on hot griddle. Serve with jam topping. Serves two.

JESSIE'S MASHED-POTATO PANCAKES

> 8 ounces leftover mashed potatoes
>
> 1 egg
>
> $\frac{1}{4}$ to $\frac{1}{2}$ cup flour (as needed)

Mix egg with potatoes, then add flour. Spoon mixture onto hot griddle to form pancakes. Serves two.

- Try custards and pudding—not only as dessert foods, but as meal substitutes or snacks.

- Puree vegetables in blender or food processor.

- Don't be embarrassed to try baby foods—or applesauce.

- Avoid elaborate sauces, but do use sauce if it gives simple foods a flavor that you can tolerate or even enjoy. Favorites reported by many patients are lemony or mustardy sauces.

- Many patients report that cold foods are easier for them to swallow. Try simple foods that have been frozen—frozen gazpacho, for example.

- Drink a milk shake with an egg blended into it—this can be a complete meal or snack.

- Soups are a meal within a bowl. Try them hot or cold—even frozen.

- Pasta seems to have therapeutic benefits. If the sauce is too spicy, try a simple sauce or merely some melted butter. Pasta can be eaten hot or cold.

Exercise

Exercise has become an important part of the American way of life and will continue to be part of your lifestyle as a patient. Whether you were a dedicated Jane Fonda Workout fan or a confirmed nonexerciser, you will find a need for exercise as part of your recovery.

Discuss exercise with your doctor. Most patients work through three stages of recovery:

1. Beginning exercises, usually geared specifically toward helping to heal a surgical wound.

2. Medium exercises, after the wound has healed and as a beginning step toward more serious exercise.

3. Strenuous exercises, which may mean a return to your pre-diagnosis exercise program.

While you are undergoing radiation or chemotherapy, you may not be strong enough for a serious exercise program. After treatment, the fatigue that is associated with interferon, chemo, and radiotherapy will abate—usually within six weeks. As you get your weight in shape and begin to feel better, exercise will become a more exciting thought. If you are used to regular exercise, you'll be anxious to get back to it. If you were not a devotee of the workout before, you may find that a three-times-a-week beginner's class helps you to recover mentally and physically from the last residues of treatment. If you suffer from depression or lack of get-up-and-go, exercise can give you new energy and serve as a vital link to your recovery.

Indeed, exercise is so important to your recovery that you will probably begin some form of exercise while you are still in the hospital. This will vary with the type of surgery you have, naturally—but don't be surprised if you are taught breathing exercises for chest surgery patients.

Walking is one of the best exercises you can ever give your body—you'll begin walking in the hospital just as an endeavor to get out of bed, build up your strength, and get out of the confines of your room. As you recover, walk farther and faster. Walking at a brisk pace can be terrific aerobic exercise and is a fabulous way to help control weight, build up endurance, and fight depression.

Postmastectomy Exercises—Beginner

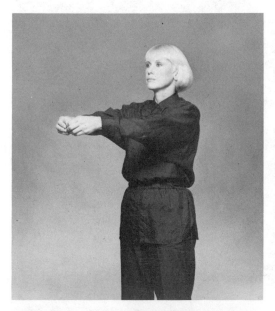

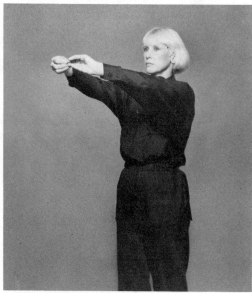

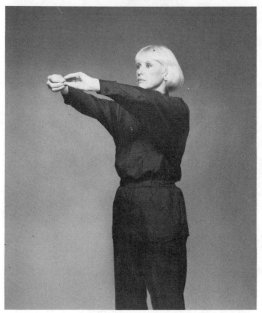

THE EENTSY WEENTSY SPIDER

1. Start with both arms outstretched in front of you (*in bed, chair, or standing*).
2. Put your fingers together as if to begin playing the Eentsy Weentsy Spider game. ("Out came the sun and dried up all the rain, and the eentsy weentsy spider went up the spout again.")

(*continued*)

3. As you move your fingers and rotate your wrists, slowly raise your arms as high as you can.
4. Drop arms and hands to your sides, relax, then begin again.
5. Build up gradually, beginning with one or two completions and working your way up to ten over the next two to three weeks.

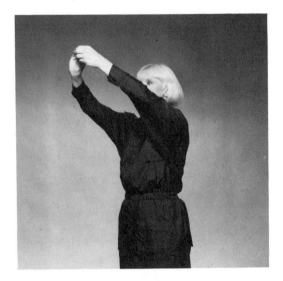

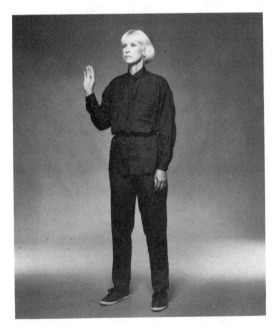

THE QUEEN ELIZABETH WAVE

1. Practice this wave (*in bed, chair, or standing*) with the arm on your surgical side; it is not necessary to wave with the other hand.
2. Bend your arm at the elbow, keeping your elbow at approximately waist level. Raise your hand up to wave in the flat motion used by Her Royal Highness.

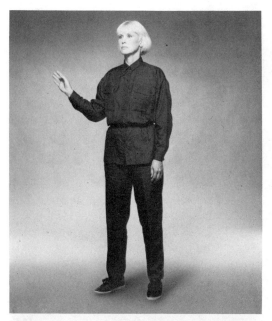

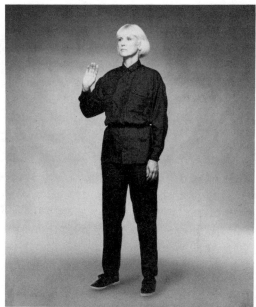

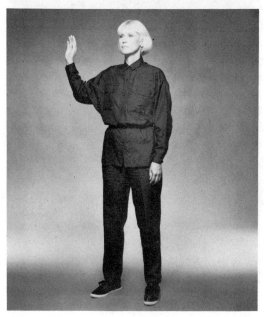

3. Wave your hand as if greeting throngs of loyal subjects—Queen Elizabeth style. This is done by moving the entire arm and hand slightly in a side-to-side motion from the wrist and elbow.
4. Wave five waves, then raise arm away from the body and wave again.
5. For the third waving sequence, move arm farther away from your body and wave to the crowds out there.
6. Wave hand five times per position. Rest after each sequence.
7. Build up to ten 3-part sequences as you recuperate.

GLORIA'S RUBBER BALL SQUEEZE

1. Using the rubber ball the volunteer from Reach for Recovery has given you, or another small rubber ball, practice this exercise (*in bed, chair, or standing*) on the side where you had surgery.
2. Stretch your arm out in front of you, palm up with ball in hand.
3. Close hand and squeeze the ball firmly.
4. While still squeezing, bring your arm toward your body so that the fist with the ball inside it touches your collarbone.

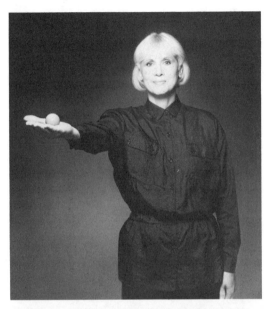

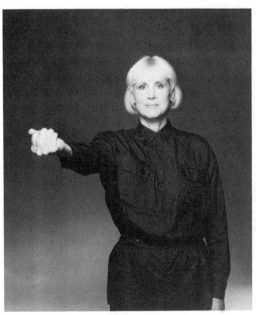

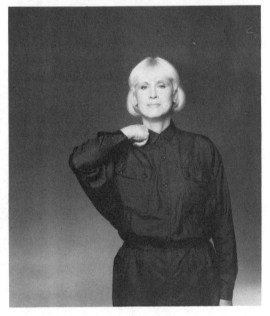

5. Stop squeezing, but keep the ball within your fist.
6. Return your arm to the original position and relax.
7. Repeat as you build up to ten.

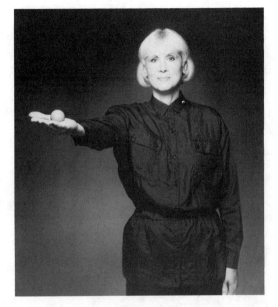

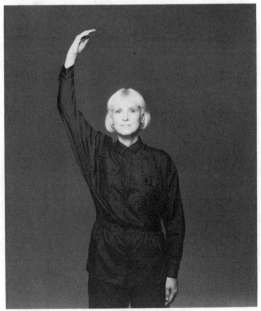

WIND IN THE WILLOW

1. Begin with arms at your sides in a relaxed position (*in bed, chair, or standing*).
2. Lift one arm sideways, away from the body and up, arching it as you reach overhead.

(*continued*)

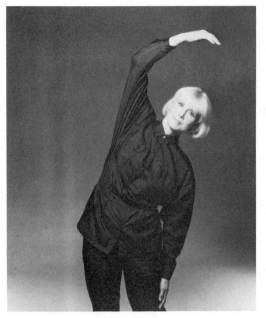
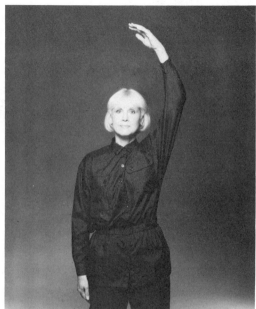

3. Move your body sideways from the waist four times as you continue to reach overhead.
4. Alternate arms and sides.
5. When you first begin this exercise, do not be alarmed if you cannot reach over your head. This will come slowly. Build up to ten sequences per side.

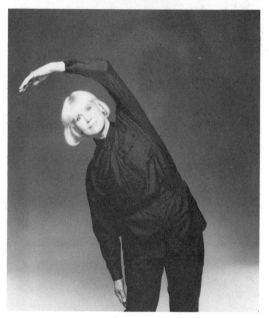

SHOULDER MOLDERS

1. Start with you hands placed on your hips (*in bed, chair, or standing*).
2. Rotate shoulders forward, moving elbows forward at the same time. This will pull a little on the side where you had surgery.
3. Do five forward, then reverse to five backward rotations. If you are in bed, sit up for these, making sure the pillows behind you do not impede movement. Rest between sets. Build up to ten full sequences.

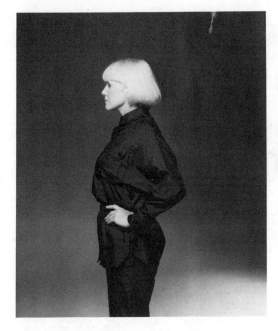
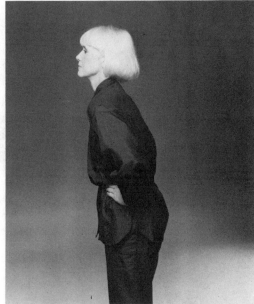

LITTLE TEAPOT

1. Put one hand on your hip (*in bed, chair, or standing—this is a little difficult in bed*), the other turned out away from your body to form a spout as you did when you were a child performing "I'm a little teapot short and stout, here is my handle, here is my spout."

2. When you get to "Tip me over and pour me out," bend at the waist to tip your spout.

3. Alternate sides. Build up to ten per side.

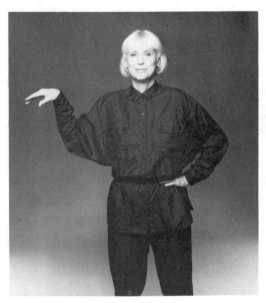 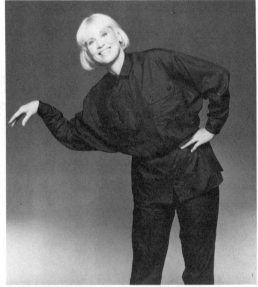

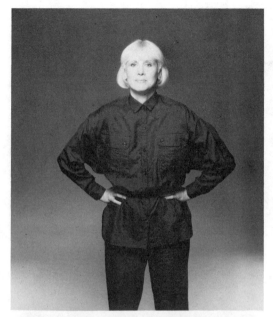

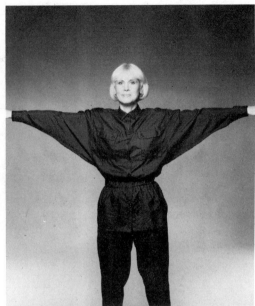

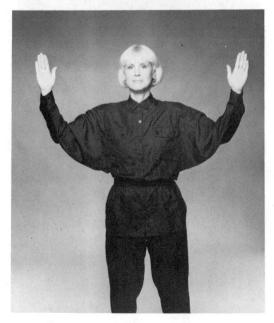

MY LORD

1. Start with your hands placed on your hips (*in bed, chair, or standing*).
2. Stretch arms out to your sides, as wide as you can.
3. Bending at the elbows, bring your hands up and together until you can press your palms together in front of your body. Pretend you are an extra in *The King and I.*

(*continued*)

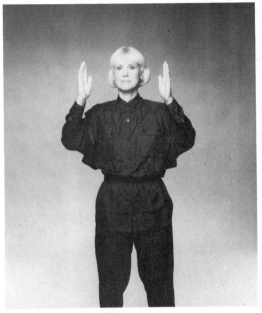

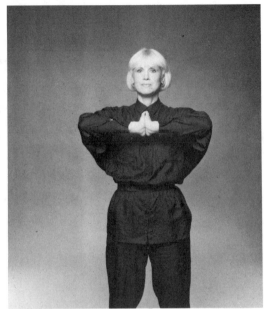

4. When your hands are palm to palm, in prayerlike position, bring your arms toward your body so that your fingertips touch your chin.
5. Bow your head, out of deference to the King of Siam, of course.
6. Rest and repeat sequence, building up to ten.

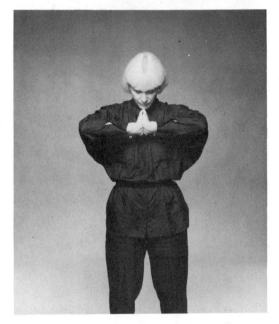

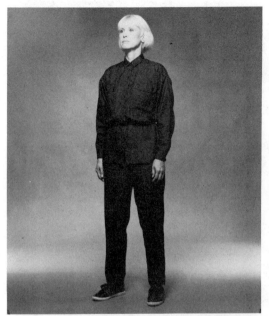

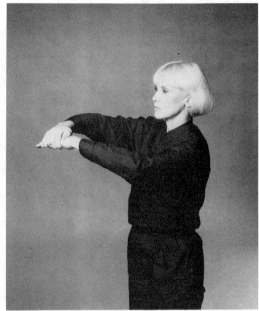

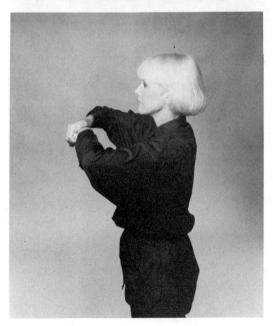

INVISIBLE-BEAR HUG

1. Begin with arms resting comfortably at your side (*in bed, chair, or standing*).
2. Reach out and arch your arms to encircle a great big invisible bear that is standing in front of you.
3. As you hug the bear, use the hand on your surgical side to clasp your other hand to firm up your grip on the bear. Make it a strong clasp, so that the bear doesn't get away.

(*continued*)

4. Bring your clasped hands closer to
   your body, progressing inward in
   three movements, hugging the bear
   closer to your body.
5. Release, relax, and repeat up to ten
   times.

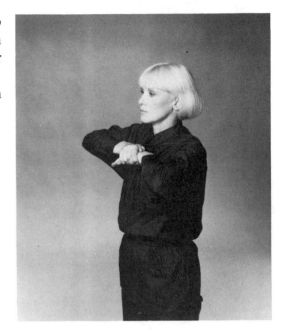

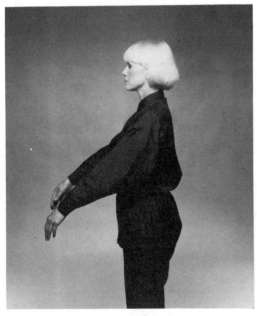

SWING LOW

1. Relax with arms at your side (*in chair
   or standing—standing is better*).
2. Swing your arms forward and then
   back to the original position, going
   slowly but increasing the momen-
   tum of the wing each time so that
   you gradually get higher.

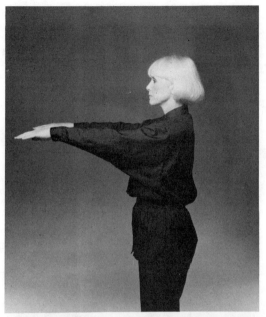

3. And higher.
4. And higher.

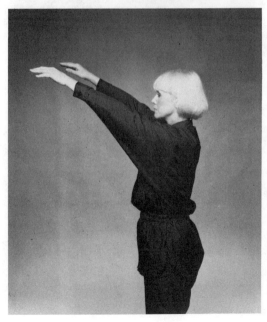

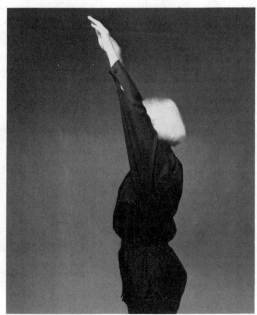

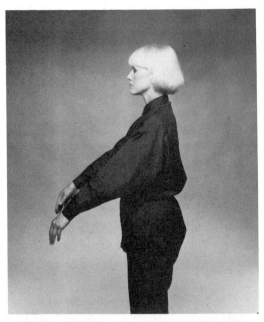

SWING LOW DOUBLE O

1. Repeat Swing Low exercise above (*standing*).

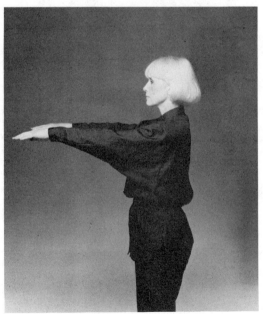

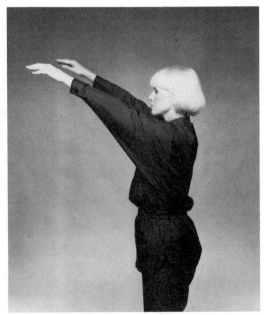

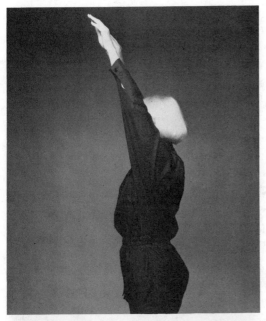

2. When your arms are as high up as you can get them—which, hopefully, is near your head—use a burst of energy and swing them backwards and around as if you were a butterfly.
3. Relax, then repeat. Work up to ten.

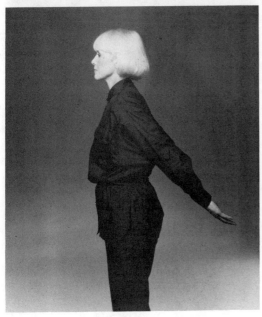

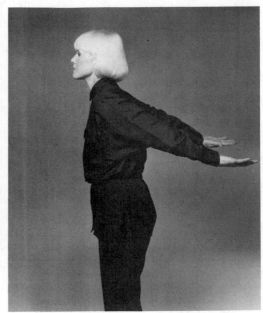

Postmastectomy Exercises—Intermediate (with Weights)

You must have your doctor's permission to work with weights after surgery. *Do not* even consider these exercises until four weeks after surgery. Use a one-pound weight on your surgical side (only) or fill a tube sock with one pound of sand and tie it off with a rubber band or plastic-bag tie. *Do not* use a heavier weight until you have been exercising for at least three weeks. Then build up gradually. *Never* use weights in bed. These exercises are to be done in a sitting or standing position.

Before you begin using your weights, warm up. You may do this with a series of exercises from the previous section for beginners. Warm up with ten minutes of mild exercises. *A warm-up is essential to your good health.*

Start each exercise with five repetitions, increasing by five each day but holding at twenty-five repetitions maximum.

MODIFIED QUEEN ELIZABETH WAVE

1. With weight in hand, bend your elbow, keeping it at waist level, and wave to the crowd as you did in the Queen Elizabeth Wave exercise.
2. Raise your hand up to wave in the flat motion used by Her Royal Highness.
3. As before, wave your hand as if greeting throngs of loyal subjects. This is done by moving the entire arm and hand slightly in a side-to-side motion from the wrist and elbow.

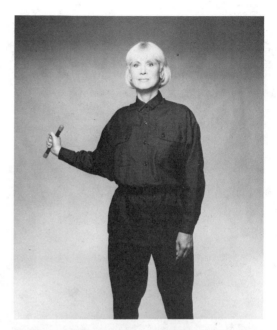

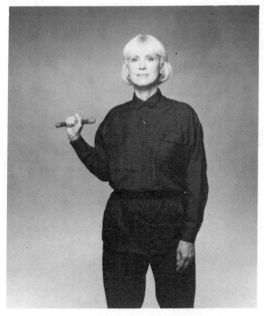

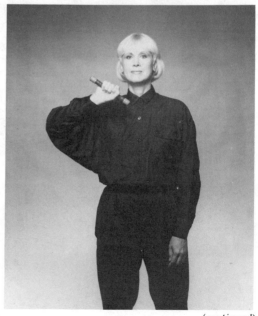

(continued)

4. Wave five times, then raise arm away from the body and wave again.
5. For the third waving sequence, move arm farther away from your body and wave to the crowds out there.
6. Wave hand five times per position. Rest after each sequence.

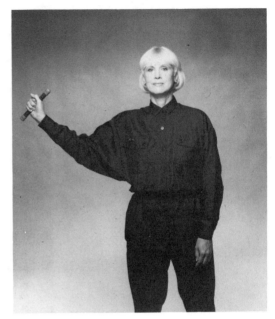

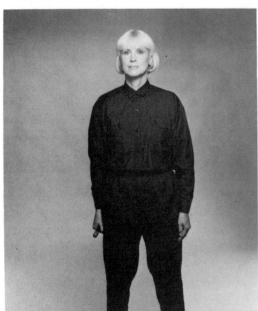

PUMP TWO

1. Relax with arms at sides, gripping weight with surgical side.

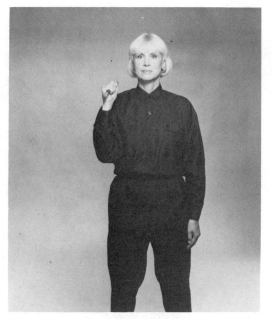

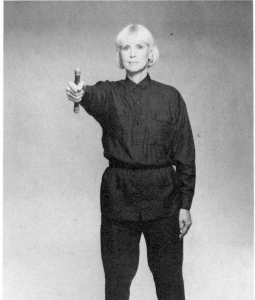

2. Bend arm at elbow and bring weighted hand up as high as you can, hopefully to shoulder level.
3. Extend arm out, with weight in hand.
4. Return to the shoulder-height position.

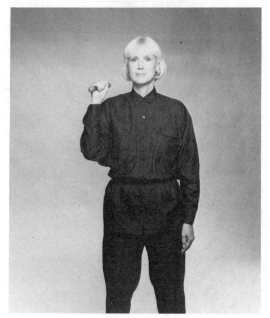

(continued)

5. Extend the arm out again, this time to the side at an angle.

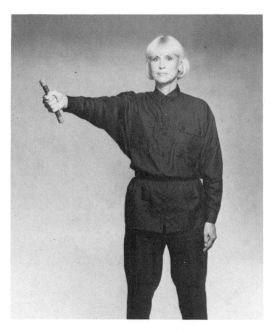

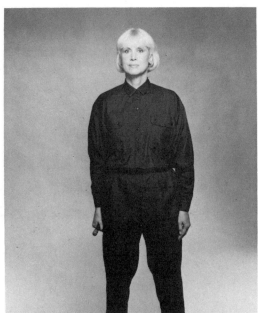

OLYMPIC GOLD

1. Relax with arms at sides, gripping weight with surgical side.

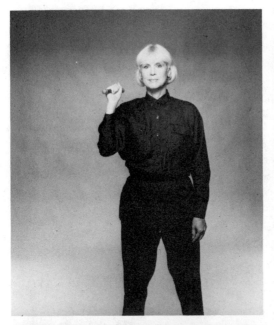

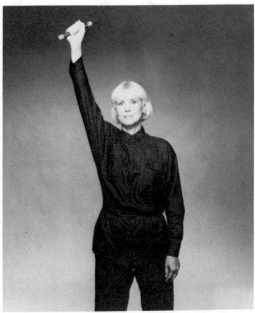

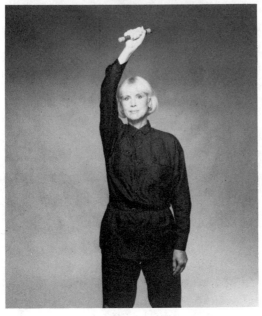

2. Raise arm as high over your head as possible. Pause, displaying the weight as if it were an Olympic gold medal that everyone wants to see. Smile for Howard Cosell.
3. Wave the gold for Mom to see.

(continued)

4. Now for the crowd. Wave in all directions while displaying the trophy.

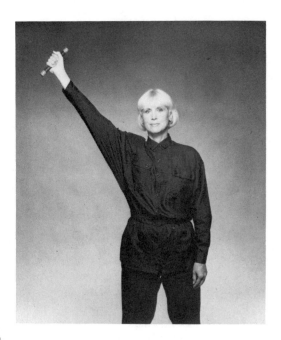

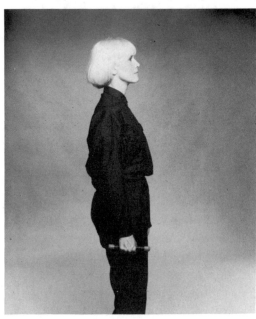

BACKWARD ARM LIFTS

1. Begin with arms at sides, gripping weight with surgical side.

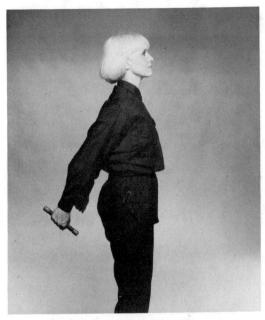

2. Pull both arms back and out behind you, raising them as high as you can. Do not bounce or pull.

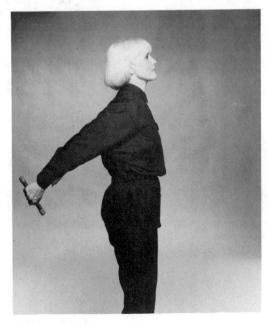

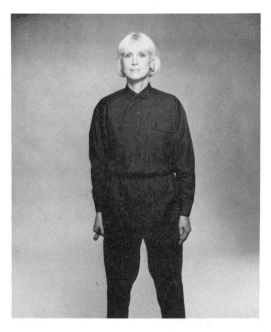

ARM HOIST

1. Begin with arms at sides, gripping weight with surgical side.
2. Raise the surgical arm by bending at the elbow, with elbow pointing to the side, and bringing your hand—with the weight—up under your armpit.

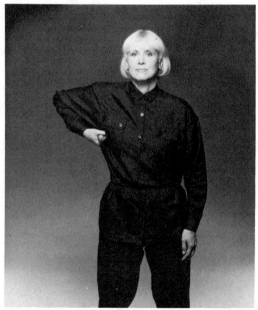

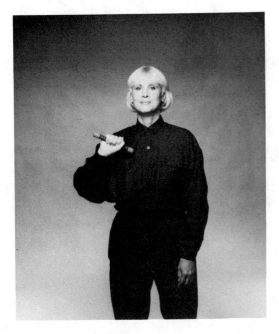

3. Lift up and out, rotating your wrist, so that the weight is now up almost at shoulder height.
4. Extend the arm while raising your hand with the weight in it.

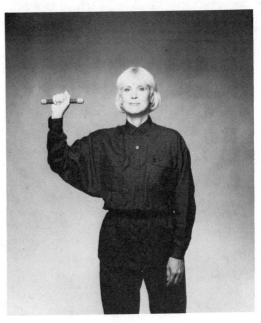

Leg Exercises

Exercising in bed is bad for your back and should not be your usual practice, especially with leg exercises. These are mild exercises that are designed to help your circulation, which is especially important after lung surgery. Your nurse will begin to exercise you automatically. *Do not* attempt an exercise program on your own without your doctor's permission and help from a nurse or nurse's aide.

Once you are able to get out of bed, if you are steady enough, lean against a chair or bed guard and do these leg exercises. Begin with five repetitions, increasing by five each day, but holding at twenty-five maximum. *Do not* do them unsupervised or without proper support. They are to aid circulation and flexibility, not to build muscles.

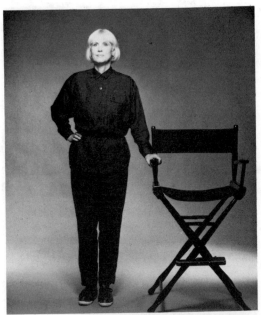

STICK 'EM UP

1. Begin by leaning on chair or bed rail.
2. Flex toes on right foot and raise right leg a few inches off the ground. Do not raise leg as high as you can; this is not an audition for the Folies-Bergère. A few inches—six to eight—is fine.
3. Return leg to ground; relax.
4. Alternate legs.

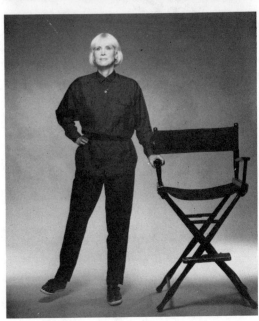

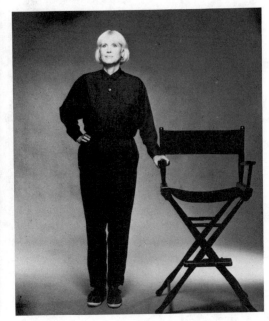

LEG SWINGS

1. Lean on chair or bed rail
2. Raise your right leg slightly off the ground and rotate or swing it out.
3. Return to beginning position.
4. Alternate legs.

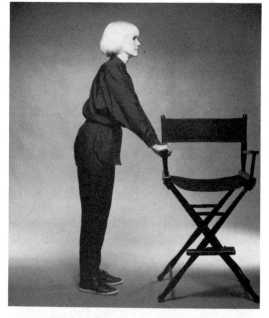

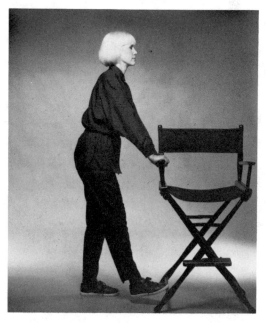

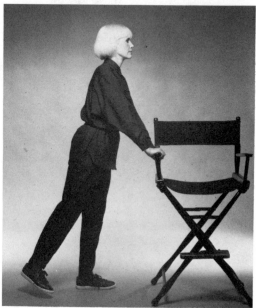

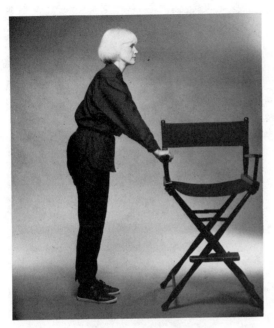

LEG BENDS

1. Lean on chair or rail.
2. Raise your right leg and bend at the knee.
3. As best you can, bring the bent leg close to your body.
4. Alternate legs.

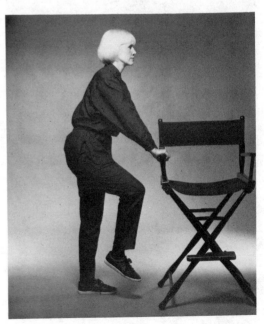

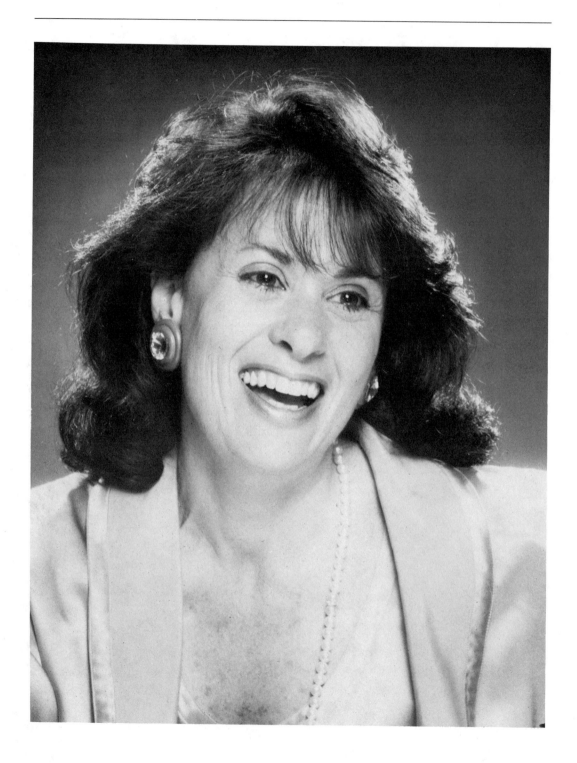

Chapter Eight

FEELING GOOD

Feelings

Very few people go through so complex a shift of feelings as cancer patients. One day you're feeling fine; the next day your world is shattered. No amount of anticipation can prepare you for the moment the doctor gives you the diagnosis.

The most important thing to remember is that although your life will change immediately, a cancer diagnosis does not mean that you are going to die; nor does it mean that after your treatment, your life can't go back to the way it was. In their terror, many patients don't see that treatment is a temporary stage. After treatment, many patients resume the lifestyle they had before diagnosis. Most patients feel changed within themselves, but their lives after treatment need not be radically changed. Many do indeed live happily ever after.

In fact, so many patients now live happily ever after that not too long ago the medical community was caught by surprise. Scientists and psychologists found their available knowledge lacking when it came to dealing with questions and support for long-term survivors. In the last few years this has been corrected, and more and more medical professionals are trained to deal with survivors. Oncologists may tell you that you have a slow-moving disease in a fast-moving field—new research, new cures, new possibilities are always around the bend. For some types of cancer, each year brings greater victories and fewer deaths.

Yet even long-term survivors are still struggling to come to grips with their feelings; some are still overwhelmed by their feelings. Some are able to verbalize their thoughts only now, many years after their trauma. Others are surprised to find they have new feelings, or are having difficulty with the realization that they really are cured.

Most patients will ride a roller coaster of emotions, beginning with "Why Me?" and moving up and down through feelings of confusion, anger, fear, self-pity, triumph, challenge, denial, and acceptance— with many others thrown in for good measure.

"My chief emotion during treatment was one of love and gratitude," says one woman. "I was so appreciative of my friends and family and all the people who turned out for me. I had never stopped to realize what good friends I had; I'd never thought about how nice people can be when you need them. They really rise to the occasion. My eyes were always filling with tears not because I was ill or afraid, but from thankfulness. It was worth getting sick to appreciate and to be able to see how beautiful the human community can be."

"I was astounded at the amount of anger I had inside me. But after the initial bout with self-pity, what shocked me was that it became positive anger. I was so mad that anything dared to invade my body and frighten my family in this manner, that I would and could give it back double trouble. With each blast of chemotherapy, as tired and sick as I felt, I had a surge of inner glory, of positive energy, that I was giving it back some of its own. I felt like this was war; this was rape. Anger was all I had to fight back with, and anger kept me going. Now I get angry when I hear other patients complain."

Some patients suffer from double-edged feelings: on one level they deal with superficial feelings, while underneath they keep another set very much in check. They feel constantly ambivalent about their condition and their course of treatment. Other patients think it's against the rules to play anything but the Good Patient game—they put on a cheerful front, tell everyone they are doing just fine, and keep their private fears in a very private place. Unfortunately, the front is so hard to keep intact that the patient resigns her true feelings to herself and takes less and less interest in her treatment and in her ability to control her situation. The Good Patient is not necessarily the happy patient.

While there may be no happy cancer patients, there are some who cope better than others. Furthermore, their positive coping techniques enhance their lives immediately. These patients bear in mind what some psychologists call the "three C's of coping": commitment, control, and challenge. The patient who copes best is committed to her recovery, wants to take some control over her treatment, and is ready to rise to the challenge of getting better.

Admitting to your feelings, no matter how crazy you think they are, is an important aspect of coping. Expressing those feelings, after you admit them to yourself, and getting information to deal with them, makes the coping process more complete. Once you have information, you can turn to family, friends, and support groups to enhance your life. Assessing your feelings, sharing them, and taking support from your inner circle are the best ways to cope with one of the most difficult periods of your life, to meet the challenge of cancer treatment.

Periods of Adjustment

Psychological studies of cancer patients show that the first year after diagnosis is the most difficult but that there are particular times during their progress toward good health at which patients are most in need of information and support:

- The first three months—The first three months are the most difficult for any patient. This includes the time of diagnosis, the time of immediate decisions (second opinions, surgery, treatments), the postoperative period (when surgery has been indicated), and the first therapy treatments.

- The end of treatment—No matter how terrible an ordeal the chemotherapy or radiotherapy has been, each patient goes through a period of psychological adjustment when she moves from a schedule of intense treatments to a maintenance program. The active attack on the disease has ceased, the wait-and-see period has begun; most patients need help in making the transition to a more normal—and eventually to their former—lifestyle. They are afraid; the adjustment can be difficult.

- The milestone years—Doctors predict a different rate of cure for differing types of cancer. After three, five, or seven years without further incidence, the doctor will pronounce you cured. While lingering fears of a recurrence haunt some patients for the rest of their lives, other patients have difficulty adjusting to the very fact that they have triumphed over the challenge. After the milestone year, some patients will reassess their lives and goals and arrive at a vision of the future that is vastly different from the one they had before they became ill. Others will count the treatment years as a mere inconvenience and may even block them out. Yet each anniversary of the cure is a special date to each cancer patient. It's not only a time to celebrate life, but a time of reflection and sometimes turmoil.

Members of the Club

Now that you have cancer, you are a member of a very elite club. You are different from other people but similar to other cancer patients; you share a bond that will separate you from the rest of society. With your diagnosis, you cross over into a world that cannot be understood by anyone who has not been in a life-threatening situation. Just as no one can *really* understand what it is like for someone else to have survived a concentration camp, a bombing, or a life of extreme poverty and hardship, no one but another cancer survivor can understand your new position in life.

To your discomfort, you will soon see that many of the social rules of the world were made by people who have not suffered; by people who have never fought for their lives or their rights and who may not have the same values you do. To protect their rules and values, they have created a barrier to shield themselves from life's more unpleasant realities—the poor and the homeless may not enter, the ill and the infirm are not welcome. Society perceives cancer as a stigma and actually makes life more difficult for the patient. Society discriminates against the cancer patient and causes silent hurt, suffering, and frustration. Only leprosy and AIDS carry greater social stigmas.

"I think that someday, in a generation or two, there will be a cancer awareness program and children will be taught about cancer," says one health education official. "Just as we now teach children the dangers of cigarette smoking, as we teach them to say 'no' to drugs—we will have to teach them that cancer is just another disease. Combating fear and misunderstanding is an educational problem."

People's misunderstanding expresses itself in various ways:

"They" don't like to hear about cancer; it frightens them.

"They" don't want to think about your problems; God forbid they should some day have the same problems.

"They" don't want to see your hair loss, or any visible sign that your life is different during treatment.

"They" think that chemotherapy is poison. We know that cancer is poison and chemotherapy is just strong medicine.

"They" think that cancer may be contagious and wonder if they should kiss you, or employ you.

"They" don't know whether you want to talk about it, so rather than ask you how you feel, they whisper behind your back.

They mean you well. But they are afraid. They are vulnerable. They do not know how to cope. They do not realize that when you become a member of the club you become an expert in coping.

Coping Strategies—
A Hero Is More Than a Sandwich

Coping traits are personal: any one person will cope with cancer in much the same way she would cope with any other crisis in her life. There is no one best way to cope, no right or wrong way—although some personalities do cope better than others. Regardless of your talents in a crisis, there are a few strategies that will help anyone in any stress situation.

Panic is the antithesis of coping. It's a disease in itself. For the cancer patient, panic can be worse than the disease. The opposite of panic may be calm, but calm can only be achieved through organization. The steps to that organization are very simple: (1) get information and (2) get help.

To enhance your coping skills, you must follow through from step one to step two. Coping, after all, is a matter of changing your behavior to fit a new set of circumstances—circumstances of stress that may not be in your personal vocabulary of normal behavior. Some philosophers say that you never really know a person until you see how they react in a crisis; the 250 episodes of the hit television show *M*A*S*H* were built on the very theme that ordinary people do extraordinary things when they reach out in a crisis. A hero is not just the person who runs off to the battlefield, but the one who can adapt her behavior to maximize her personal strengths in the time of crisis.

Coping is a compromise position. If you had your choice, you wouldn't be in the crisis situation in the first place. But your only choice now is how well you can adapt; how well you can turn this new situation around so that it works for you instead of against you.

Information Please

The first step in coping is to get more information about your personal situation. You must do this whether you are in an earthquake, on the highway alone with a flat tire, or at home contemplating your cancer diagnosis. Sure, you can cry, panic, or feel sorry for yourself if you want to. But these will not be appropriate responses until you really know what your situation is. As soon as you are able, hopefully as early as your first visits with your doctors, start asking for information. Remember, there is no such thing as a stupid question.

It is a common phenomenon that the patient forgets everything the doctor tells her at the first meeting. Patients walk out of the doctor's office with the understanding that they have cancer, but often know little more. Sometimes they are too embarrassed to tell their doctors they don't remember; sometimes they are too shy to say they didn't understand the technical or medical explanation. Very often, the patient begins to withdraw from the process of caring for her body at that very first meeting. She doesn't understand what the doctor says; the mention of drug names and medical terms sounds confusing and impossible to learn; she assigns her care to her doctor and complacently becomes the Good Patient. The Good Patient is afraid to ask too many questions, to take up too much of the doctor's time, to appear "dumb," to rock the boat, or to question treatments. Sometimes the Good Patient doesn't even want to ask for a second opinion, for fear of hurting the doctor's feelings. While patients of both sexes suffer from the Good Patient complex, it is an easier role for women to assume because they not only feel weak and threatened by the disease and the uncertainty of their future but have generations of prior behavioral learning that tells them to defer to a big, strong man who will make it all better—a doctor.

One study of patient involvement and cure rate used the names of chemotherapy drugs as the test variable. The patients who did not take the time or trouble, and did not have the curiosity to learn the names of the drugs they were taking were contrasted to a group of patients who knew the names of every drug they were taking, and often knew the dosage and the rotation schedule. The patients who knew the names of the drugs had a higher survival rate.

The truly good patient wants to participate in her treatment and her recovery. Not only does she learn her drugs but she learns as much as she can about her situation. Some patients go to medical school libraries and read the latest papers on their condition. Others go to university bookstores and buy basic books on cancer—handbooks and guidebooks on drugs and treatments, written for physicians and students. Others go to libraries (you usually need a specialized library for specific information about cancer) or talk to outside doctors, not only to get another opinion on their condition but to hear possible procedures and learn the range of treatment options.

Information helps alleviate feelings of anxiety and stress; it makes the patient better able to prepare her actions. It is important, however, that all the information not come from one source. While your doctor now plays a critical role in your recovery, he should not be your only source of information. Use several sources and then trust yourself to sort out what you've learned. Much of what you read will be contradictory. Discuss the contradictions with your doctors and nurses and get their opinions. Use common sense; don't swallow anyone's theories until you have digested them.

"My doctor seemed to withhold information from me," says one woman. "It wasn't that he wasn't telling me the truth about my condition, or my changes, as he kept saying that he just didn't know, or he said that every patient reacted differently. He could give me statistics, but if I was going to be the one in one thousand who got blisters on my tongue—that was clearly a variable. I found the best information

I got came from other cancer patients. Patients are much more willing to tell you good and bad things than doctors are. Besides, in the back of your mind is a denial process going on that says, 'Well, even if most patients lose their hair, I won't, I'll be the 3 percent...' or whatever it is that your doctor tells you."

"Patients have to realize that they can be part of the process. Doctors are only human. They're taking a lot of calculated risks. If you want to know what their calculations are, you have to know enough about the subject to ask good questions, to show your doctor you care enough about your body and what he plans to do to it. If you're not well enough to go to the library and get a lot of books, have someone do this for you. People always want to do something to help you. Learning is something that helps. And get lots of different opinions. And learn a lot of odds, so you know where you want to take risks and where you don't. Having cancer can teach you a lot about risk taking, but you can only do it if you get smart."

A study conducted in the Netherlands compared breast cancer patients with Hodgkin's disease patients to study their affiliation behavior. Those patients who took the time to seek help from their fellow sufferers felt a reduction in stress and felt their coping was made more successful by the help and support they received. Both sets of patients were troubled by uncertainty about the origin of their disease; both sets of patients solved this anxiety by obtaining direct information about their form of cancer. Questions about survival rates and side effects of treatment were also answered through direct information sources. But the patients who were concerned about how to get help, what to do to help prevent future illness, and how to solve practical, social, and psychological problems found their information through contact with other patients. Furthermore, the study found that the person who was more likely to reach out to a fellow sufferer to talk had better coping skills and was not inclined to "give up" in a stressful situation.

By comparing themselves to people in the same situation, cancer patients can come to their own, more personal, conclusions. What's "normal" comes to be defined by the closed society; it is for the members of the club to decide what feelings and reactions are "socially acceptable."

Therefore the information a cancer patient needs comes in two forms—hard information, or book learning, and soft information, which comes by word of mouth and may or may not be as accurate as hard information, although its social implications may be more comforting.

Talking It Out

Often the getting of information is a verbal process. Certainly working with other cancer patients is a verbal process. But information cannot just come in; it must also go out. Being able to ask questions, express feelings, and let off steam are important parts of the communication process. Talking it out is the bridge between getting information and being able to use it to your best advantage.

The talking process affects not only the patient herself, but her inner circle—spouse, family, friends. All members of the team need to talk and to communicate. Then the inner circle can decide how best to approach the outer circle—how to talk to friends who are not so close, to employers, to new acquaintances.

Talking it out means listening and hearing what the other person has to say. This is not a time to make assumptions, to take another person for granted, or to second-guess anyone's intentions. The patient who is best able to verbalize her feelings and make her needs clear to those around her will be able to make a functioning support group of her inner circle. The patient who sends out coded messages, who fakes feelings for lack of knowing what to do or what to say, who adapts certain behavior patterns because she is unable to deal with her true situation, is only getting in the way of her own recovery—which isn't, by the way, an unusual circumstance.

Out of fear, many people do not say what they really want or even allow themselves to think about what they really want. Sometimes they want to give up all responsibility for their care—mental as well as physical responsibility. They retreat into a never-never land and dare their close ones to try to reach them. If you identify with this behavior, realize that it is common and know that you are not alone. Seek counseling with an oncological nurse or psychologist who can put you on the track toward getting in touch with your real feelings. Sometimes it's easier to talk to a stranger than to your closest relative because you are so afraid, and are doubly afraid that your fears will upset your family and make matters worse. Most families come through the crisis better than the patient expects them to, but your family can only be helpful when you communicate your wants and needs to them.

Support Systems

Once your feelings have come out in the open, you are ready to develop your own support system. There are now organized support systems in the form of medical, community, religious, and special interest groups. However, your main support group will most likely be your inner circle. The use you make of this support system will be a critical factor in how well you cope with your illness and treatment and how well you recover.

Numerous psychological studies of cancer patients have shown that patients who reach out for help and accept it end up coping better with their situation and improving the quality of their life. Some patients try to shut out their families either by directly denying that they are in need or by behaving in a way that intentionally cuts people off and distances them. Those who accept the fact that treatment will temporarily—or even permanently—cause them to slow down, lose some control over their bodies, and live by a new set of rules are the ones who adjust most quickly to the changes caused by diagnosis.

In a recent study reported in *Cancer* (January 1986), clinicians created a support group to reduce the psychological difficulties of patients and assess the long-term benefits of thematic counseling. Women with gynecologic cancer received eight counseling sessions focused on information about cancer, progressive relaxation, diet, and exercise. The women who received the counseling were significantly less depressed and less anxious than a control group of noncounseled patients and reported greater knowledge of their illness, better relationships with caregivers, fewer sexual difficulties, and more participation in leisure activities. The study's results can be applied to individual counseling or group counseling and to other varieties of cancer.

Another study, this one at King's College Hospital in London, showed that individual counseling was slightly more effective than group counseling. Individual counseling, it was felt, better enabled the patient to vent her private emotions and to draw on her own resources to cope and adjust. The study further showed that patients who had been counseled were significantly more likely to report greater personal control over their lives than noncounseled patients three months after surgery. At twelve months after surgery, the control group and the counseled group scored more similarly in their reporting of problems and experiences.

In another study at the same hospital, patients were encouraged to seek counseling, which was provided for free; the mean number of sessions requested was six. These sessions were generally held between the immediate preoperative and the postoperative period.

The moral of the story is simple: counseling seems to help a tremendous number of women. Often counseling sessions are free, but even if they are not, they appear to be a worthwhile investment. Even if the sessions cost as much as $100 each, this $600—which your health plan should cover—can make the difference in how you feel for the first year after diagnosis and perhaps for the rest of your life.

Support brings comfort, helps to alleviate fear and anxiety, strengthens feelings of control, and increases self-esteem. Although most patients report that their primary source of support is their spouse, they also count their other family members, friends, nurses, and organized support groups as part of their recovery team. In a Dutch study, only one in four patients considered the doctor an important support figure. Also one in four reported that they obtained important support from one or more fellow sufferers.

If you find that your inner circle is too confused or hurt to offer the kind of support you need (this is not uncommon), talk to your oncological nurse. There are counseling groups for the whole family that will teach members how to become a functioning support group. Cancer is a family illness. Everyone should seek information to be better able to cope; everyone should get counseling and be part of a greater support network.

The Buddy System

For many people, accepting the need for support is difficult. They hate the idea that they are now dependent on others for their care and comfort and often prefer to be uncomfortable rather than burden someone.

Some studies have shown that one of the cancer patient's most dreaded fears is loss of independence. These patients have forgotten about the buddy system.

The buddy system, developed for child safety in swimming pools, assigns each child a buddy who is in some way responsible for the other's well-being. In most cases, the buddy is not able to assume true responsibility but functions within the psychological realm of a tiny support system. During a "buddy check," buddies are to seek each other out, grasp hands, and raise them to be counted.

Cancer patients who are undergoing therapy must also accept the buddy system as an integral part of the recovery process. Just as every woman using natural childbirth techniques has a coach, every chemo patient needs a buddy. The buddy need not be a spouse; it need not be the same person every day or every week. The buddy just needs to be in the swimming pool at the time of that particular chemotherapy session.

The buddy's job is to drive her friend to her treatment and to sit with her and wait for the treatment, and then drive to her home. She offers aid, companionship, a listening ear, and a hand to hold—as needed. Often patients must wait for long periods of time even when they have specific appointments. During this time they can get lonely, depressed, or merely bored. Although most patients bring books, magazines, knitting, or needlework, they still feel better when they have a companion. Anticipation of the treatment may cause anxiety. The buddy is there to be driver, listener, babysitter, and friend. While some outpatients are reluctant to ask someone to drive them to treatment sessions, few should be allowed to drive themselves. Members of the inner circle should organize a functioning buddy system if they are unable to be on hand for each treatment.

Each patient needs a buddy; each buddy needs to understand the intimate nature of the relationship.

Taking Responsibility

About one-third of all cancer patients move into a passive role after diagnosis and feel that their situation is beyond their control. The remaining patients believe they can affect the outcome of their illness. They want to participate actively in getting better, and in many cases they want to take back control of their lives from doctors and medical machines. Some people want to have a part in the medical decisions that are made; some merely want the freedom to refuse certain (or even all) treatments.

Taking responsibility means not only learning the facts about your illness and its treatment, but planning ahead to your recovery period when you can effect more positive changes in your body. If you still smoke, stop now. Improve your diet and exercise programs. Cut down on drinking. Work to make your body work better so that it is well tuned and you are in tune with it. Knowing your body well will help you identify future problems if they ever arise.

Knowing that hard information (facts) and soft information (support) combine to cut down on the stresses of the cancer patient, you must take responsibility for gaining access. Don't count on information coming to you—go after it. You must actively seek information and share it with your inner circle. Personal feelings of control will also be enhanced when you do something to help yourself.

No matter how much other people show themselves willing to do for you, the first steps are yours alone. Open your mind to the realities of your new situation, take responsibility for them, and you will not be without power. Being sick means losing some control, but you do not have to relinquish total control of your life. Cancer provides unique aggressiveness training. Take advantage of it.

Positive Denial

The opposite of taking control is denial. While some amount of denial is natural, especially in new patients, who often think, "This can't really be happening to me," there are other aspects of denial that can work in the patient's favor. While total denial of the realities of one's life is a sign of mental instability, selective denial has become a good coping device for some patients. Selective denial is positive denial.

Some patients are aware of the facts of their illness or treatment, but selectively ignore those that they find inconvenient. They push on with their lives, doing very much what they want to do, not denying that they are sick but denying that they are crippled. There is a huge difference.

A number of research studies have suggested that selective denial used as a coping device frequently has positive adaptive consequences. Selective deniers are more optimistic than other patients; they return to work more quickly, have fewer sexual problems, and suffer less from illness. They also suffer less from stress, and since stress can be as debilitating as any other disease-related problem, selective denial can be considered part of the recovery process.

"I call it the power of positive thinking," says one patient. "I weigh what the doctors have told me about my capabilities, what I should and shouldn't do, and then think about how much I want to do something. I limit my goals—being sick teaches you limits and priorities—so that when I accomplish a goal I feel proud that I did it, but my goal is not the same goal I might have had for myself before I was sick. I don't deny that I have a problem, but I want to deny it on a daily basis."

Selective denial also helps buy a patient more time to think through her real situation and decide what to do. Scarlett O'Hara's famous coping device—"I won't think about that today, tomorrow is another day"—is a perfect example. Each day she buys herself gives her more time to come to grips with the actual problem.

Antidepression Treatment

Health specialists have long been intrigued by the relationship between depression and cancer: Are cancer patients more depressed than other people because they have every reason to be more depressed, or are they simply more depressed because many of the drugs used to treat cancer cause depression? Researchers have a hard time distinguishing between justifiable unhappiness and serious depression.

Although not all patients complain of depression, enough suffer from this problem that doctors, nurses, and psychologists have developed various programs to help alleviate the symptoms. If you feel depressed, if you suffer from serious mood swings, if you have trouble sleeping or concentrating, talk to your nurse or doctor about it. There are a handful of different treatments which can improve your situation. The quality of your life during treatment ought to be of major concern to your doctor.

Drug Treatment: Most patients who complain of depression are asked to try mood-elevating or mood-regulating drugs. A large number of the patients who use these drugs find relief in this method of depression therapy and are satisfied with the results. But some patients just don't like the idea of taking drugs, so they seek alternative techniques.

Laugh Therapy: Norman Cousins prescribed his own laugh therapy— he made audio cassettes of his favorite comics' albums and listened to them whenever he could, especially during treatments. Studies made in the 1950s proved that joking under stress is a common coping mechanism and a useful form of defensive behavior. Don't worry about silly or "sick" jokes—just laugh. The more you laugh, the less you cry.

ReT: ReT is relaxation training—its techniques can be self-taught or learned in formal, individualized sessions. They include finding a quiet space, breathing deeply, and blocking out thoughts or problems with self-hypnosis. (Read the best-selling book *The Relaxation Response* for how-to information.) The benefits associated with ReT have been an improved mental state, better sleeping habits, greater tolerance for chemotherapy, and a minimized need for antidepressant drugs and for pain killers.

Visualization: As for ReT, training in visualization, also known as "imaging," techniques can be formal or informal. Some people read books or take lessons, others just understand the principle and adapt it to their own needs. The patient is asked to focus her powers of concentration and energy on imagining (or visualizing) the destruction of either immediate pain or specific cancer cells. You see a cancer cell in your mind's eye, and then you visualize your own white blood cells devouring it. Or the patient can be asked to use this same power to transport herself from a hospital filled with tubes and medicines to a more comfortable situation, such as an island paradise. It's clearly a case of mind over matter.

Religion

Many patients try to come to grips with their illness either by finding a religious reason for it or by taking strength from the solace their religion affords. Many patients, and their families, report a return to religion—either the religion of their childhood or a different religion which now offers comfort—and most perceive religion as another positive method of coping.

Most religions have clergy members who will visit you in the hospital, who are adept at listening to your problems, and who may be able to reinforce the links of your support groups if you are having communication problems.

Getting Better

To most people, feeling better and getting better are connected in physical and psychological ways. The process of recovery can be long and hard. There can be setbacks. Some days are better than others; some cycles are better than others. Illness teaches us to change the way we look at ourselves, our lives, and our triumphs. It is a very harsh lesson in the realities of the human condition.

"In the beginning," says a patient, "I used to pray for a miracle. A big miracle. Like I would be cured and none of this was real. Then I came to realize that every day is a miracle. And I was just too busy running around with my kids and my work and all my errands to have ever realized it until I became sick."

"You have to stop and smell the flowers," Marvella Bayh used to tell her friends.

The process of getting better remains one of small steps, taken with the greatest of care. The triumphs go to those who are willing to see them in between the cracks of pain and frustration. There is no doubt that your attitude very much affects your health and your ability to recover. Whether you have to goad yourself through every difficult day by chasing a carrot on a stick (offer yourself a reward for getting through each chemo session), or whether you use selective denial to get you up on your feet and back into the mainstream—it doesn't matter. Do what works for you. If plan B doesn't cut it, try plan C. Coping is adapting. Adapting is being able to change. When you're flexible, you'll find a new freedom. When you're committed to getting better, you are challenged by each new day. The future is what you make of it.

Makeup Shopping List

List names of colors and brands of your regular cosmetics. If you need supplies, give the shopping list to a family member or friend.

Moisturizer: _____   Foundation: _____
_____   _____
_____   _____
_____   _____

Cream blush: _____   Powder blush: _____
_____   _____
_____   _____
_____   _____

Other blush products: _____   Eye makeup: _____
_____   _____
_____   _____
_____   _____

Makeup remover: _____
_____
_____
_____

Other items: _____
_____
_____
_____

Personal Resource List and Phone Numbers

As you begin your quest for the beauty supplies and prosthetic devices you will need in order to restore your looks, fill in the names and phone numbers of, and any special notes about, the community resources you discover. Get friends to make recommendations; evaluate the information and the availability of goods and services. This will come in handy if you have questions, need refills or repairs, or want to help out another woman.

Wigs: _____

_____

_____

_____

Eyebrows: _____

_____

_____

_____

Eyelashes: _____

_____

_____

_____

Makeup: _____

_____

_____

_____

Camouflage, theatrical, or special makeup: _____

_____

_____

_____

Prosthetics: _____

_____

_____

_____

Mastectomy clothing and items from specialty shops: _____

_____

_____

_____

Ask Your Doctor

One of the most frequent problems a patient has is the inability to remember the questions she was planning on asking her doctor at their next meeting. Although your doctor probably answers some questions on the phone, use this space to write down questions for your next visit. (You may also want to read this book with a marking pen in hand. Mark the sections that you have further questions about, then write down the page numbers on this page.)

Resource List

Cancer Information Service

The Cancer Information Service is a free service designed to answer your questions. While volunteers are more adept with medical than cosmetic answers, give them a call whenever you have a question. In the United States the master number, if no number exists for your area (or you get no answer), for twenty-four-hour help is: (800) 638–6694.

Alabama: (800) 292–6201

Alaska: (800) 638–6070

California: (800) 252–9066

Colorado: (800) 332–1850

Connecticut: (800) 922–0824

Delaware: (800) 523–3586

District of Columbia: (202) 636–5700

Florida: (800) 432–5953

Georgia: (800) 327–7332

Hawaii (Oahu): 524–1234
    Other islands—ask operator for
    Enterprise 6702

Illinois: (800) 972–0586
    Chicago: (312) 226–2371

Kentucky: (800) 432–9321

Maine: (800) 225–7034

Maryland: (800) 492–1444

Massachusetts: (800) 952–7420

Minnesota: (800) 582–5262

Montana: (800) 525–0231

New Hampshire: (800) 225–7034

New Jersey: (800) 223–1000

New Mexico: (800) 525–0231

New York: (800) 462–7255
    New York City: (212) 794–7982

North Carolina: (800) 672–0943

North Dakota: (800) 328–5188

Ohio: (800) 282–6522

Pennsylvania: (800) 822–3963

Puerto Rico: (800) 638–6070

South Dakota: (800) 328–5188

Texas: (800) 392–2040
    Houston: (713) 792–3245

Vermont: (800) 225–7034

Virgin Islands: (800) 638–6070

Washington: (800) 552–7212;
    Seattle (206) 284–7263

Wisconsin: (800) 362–8038

Wyoming: (800) 525–0231

Support and Information Groups

American Cancer Society
90 Park Avenue
New York, NY 10017

(Provides support, information, and medical and financial resources; has many separate programs, such as I Can Cope, Reach for Recovery, and People Against Cancer. Has offices in major cities all over the United States.)

American Society of Plastic and Reconstructive Surgeons
233 North Michigan Avenue
Suite 1900
Chicago, IL 60601
(312) 856–1834

(Will provide a free booklet on reconstruction and the names of three board-certified surgeons in your area.)

Cancer Hopefuls United in Mutual Support (CHUMS)
3310 Rochambeau Avenue
New York, NY 10467

(Provides support groups.)

Corporate Angel Network (CAN)
(914) 328–1313

(Call 8:30 A.M. to 4:30 P.M. EST to arrange free rides on corporate airplanes for specialized cancer treatment.)

Encore

(Provides support groups. Contact your local YWCA.)

Fred Hutchinson Cancer Research Center
Medical Oncology Unit Dietary Department
Seattle, WA 98104

(Supplies free menus and dietary information for chemotherapy and radiotherapy patients.)

Leukemia Society of America
211 East 43d Street
New York, NY 10017
(212) 573–8484

(Has chapters in over fifty cities; provides aid—including financial—to patients.)

Make Today Count
P.O. Box 303
Burlington, IA 52601

(Provides family and peer support groups.)

Reach for Recovery

(Provides support groups for breast cancer patients. Contact your local American Cancer Society chapter.)

Share
(212) 228–3064

(Provides hotline to answer questions; will return your call—collect, outside the area—within twenty-four hours.)

United Ostomy Association
2001 West Beverly Boulevard
Los Angeles, CA 90057
(213) 413–5510

(Provides literature, conventions, and organized support.)

Vital Options
3960 Laurel Canyon Boulevard
(mailing address only)
Studio City, CA 91604
(818) 508–5657

(Provides support groups for patients aged 16 to 40.)

Beauty Supplies

There is usually at least one well-stocked beauty supply store in every community. Frends, the largest in Hollywood, is considered one of the best-stocked in the United States and is where most of the entertainment industry supplies are bought. It is especially good for eyebrows, eyelashes, and camouflage makeup. They will mail-order.

Frends Beauty Supply
5202 Laurel Canyon Boulevard
North Hollywood, CA 91604
(818) 769–3834

Turbans

Regalia
Palo Verde and 33d Streets
P.O. Box 27800
Tucson, AZ 85726

Wigs

Alkin Hair Company
264 West 40th Street
New York, NY 10018
(212) 719–3070

(Does weaving, braiding, extensions matched to samples.)

Allen-Arthur/Wigs of France
P.O. Box 6575
Minneapolis, MN 55406
(800) 424–7547

(Carries wigs, hairpieces, eyebrows, special chemo wigs.)

American Afro Hair Center
74 West 38th Street
New York, NY 10018
(212) 764–5546

(Specializes in Afro styles.)

Jacques Darcel
50 West 57th Street
New York, NY 10024
(212) 753–7576

(Boutique. Has large selection, private
booths.)

DeMeo Brothers Hair, Inc.
39 West 28th Street
New York, NY 10011
(212) 679–9727

(Specializes in sample matching/Euro-
pean human hair.)

Eva Gabor International
765 South Harvard Avenue
Los Angeles, CA 90005
(213) 383–2871

(Specializes in wigs, hairpieces, chemo
wigs.)

Edith Imre
8 West 56th Street
New York, NY 10024
(212) 758–0233

(Specializes in chemo wigs and related
hair problems.)

Jacquelyn Wigs
c/o Catalogs U.S.A.
P.O. Box 23039
Rochester, NY 14692

Lugo Hair Center, Ltd.
927 Flatbush Avenue
Brooklyn, NY
(718) 284–0370

(Specializes in Afro and European styles.)

Prosthetics for Hair Loss
174 Fifth Avenue
New York, NY 10011
(212) 206–6785

(Specializes in wigs for chemotherapy,
head trauma, and alopecia patients.)

René of Paris
15551 Cabrito Road
Van Nuys, CA 91406
(818) 376–1300

(Specializes in wigs for the entertainment
industry, chemotherapy patients; carries
fun wigs; does sample matching by mail.)

Patient Diary

Patient Diary

Patient Diary

Patient Diary

Index

Actinomycin D, 84
Adapting (*see* Adjustment)
Adenocarcinoma, lung, 127
Adjustment:
    adapting in, 231
    hair loss and, 34–35
    periods of, 217–218
    state of readiness for change and, 12–13
Adolfo wigs, 47, 54
Adriamycin:
    hair loss and, 31
    skin and, 84
Albolene cleansing cream, 87, 102
Alcoholic beverages, 142
Alkin Hair Company, 237
Allen-Arthur wigs, 47, 237
Allergy, 87
Alopecia, 19
    (*See also* Hair loss)
Aluminum chloride, 155
Ambivalence, 216
American Afro Hair Center, 238
American Cancer Society, 236
American Society of Plastic and
    Reconstructive Surgeons, 236
Anger, 216
Ankles, swollen, 134
Anticancer drugs (*see* Chemotherapy)
Antidepression treatment, 228–229
Antiperspirants, 155
Appearance, 3–13
    baseline checkup and, 7–8
    cancer treatment and, 9–12
    personal reactions and, 3–4
    readiness for change and, 12–13
    value of, 5–7
Aquaphor, 85, 86
Arm hoist exercise, 208–209

Asking your doctor, 220–223, 234
Asteatotic eczema, 85
Astringents, 102
Asymmetry, 94, 156
Athlete's foot, 134
Attitudes, 3–4
    and acceptance of diagnosis, 12–13
    toward cancer, 218–219
    toward hair loss, 26–28
Aveenobar, 86
Aversions to food, 178–179

Bacillus Calmette-Guérin (BCG), 11
Backward arm lift exercise, 206–207
Baldness, 37–38, 62–63
    (*See also* Hair loss)
Ball squeeze exercise, 153–154, 188–189
Barber for crew cuts, 27
Barielle cream, 132
Basal cell carcinoma, 93
    eyes and, 116–117
Baseline beauty checkup, 7–8
    skin cancer and, 89
    (*See also* Appearance)
Bath oil, 85
Bathing, 85
Beautician for crew cuts, 27
Beauty checkup, baseline, 7–8
    skin cancer and, 89
    (*See also* Appearance)
Beauty supplies source, 237
Beginner's wig, 23–24, 51–54
Beret, 71, 72
Betty Rollin trick, 159
Birth control pills, 155
Birthmarks, 93–94
Bladder cancer, 167, 168

Blasco theatrical makeup, 91
Bleaching, tooth, 137
Bleomycin, 84–85
Bloating, 180–181
Blusher, 98–99, 101–102, 105
Bob Mackie trick, 158–159
Body image, 156–157
  (*See also* Appearance)
Bonding for tooth, 137
Booster therapy, 151
Bovine collagen, 90
Bowel cancer, 167
Bowel movements, 177, 180–181
  ostomies and, 167–170
Brassieres, 154, 155, 157
Breast cancer, 148
  fears of, 146–147
  openness about, 145
  recovery from, 152–156
  treatments for, 148–152
  (*See also* Mastectomy)
Breast lumps, 147
Breast pads, covered, 158–159
Breast prosthesis, 157–162
  cost of, 161–162
  homemade, 158–159
  marketing of, 159–162
  prescriptions for, 161–162
  purchase of, 159–162
  questions to ask about, 161
  types of, 158
Breast reconstruction, 162–166
  cost of, 164
  implant scars and, 152
  nipples and, 166
  timing of, 164–166
Breast surgery, 148–150
  adjustments after, 156–157
  alternatives in, 150–151
  avoiding complications after, 155
  exercise after, 153–154, 183–209
    beginning, 185–189
    intermediate, 200–209
  preventive, 167
  prosthesis after (*see* Breast prosthesis)
  reconstruction in (*see* Breast reconstruction)
  recovery from, 152–156
Breasts, 146–167
  cancer of (*see* Breast cancer)
  lumps in, 147
  openness of discussion of, 145
  physiology of, 147
  surgery of (*see* Breast surgery)
Brown spots, camouflage of, 100

Buddy system, 225–226
Busulfan, 84

Calorie counting, 180
Camouflage makeup, 90–92
Cancer:
  bladder and bowel, 167, 168
  breast (*see* Breast cancer)
  eye, 116–118
  gynecologic, 170–171
  head and neck, 127–128
  lung, 126–127
  oral, 142–143
  skin, 92–94
    eyes and, 116–117
  social stigma of, 218
Cancer Hopefuls United in Mutual Support
  (CHUMS), 236
Cancer Information Service, 235
Cancer patients:
  buddy system and, 225–226
  cancer diagnosis and emotions of, 215–217
  involvement in own treatment, 221–223
  taking responsibility for illness outcome,
    226–227
  (*See also* Support; Support groups)
Cancer treatment, 9–12
  vitamins and, 179
  (*See also* Treatment; *specific cancer and specific
    treatment*)
Caps:
  pookey, 63–70
  ski, 74
Carcinoma:
  basal cell, 93, 116–117
  squamous cell, 93, 116–117
    lung, 127
  (*See also* Cancer)
Cellophanes, 76
Chemokit, 95
Chemosurgery, oral cancer and, 143
Chemotherapy, 9–10
  breast cancer, 152
  eyeball cancer, 117
  food aversions and, 178–179
  hair care before, 20–24
  hair loss and (*see* Hair loss)
  oral cancer, 143
  skin and, 83–89
  weight gain and, 174–175
  wounds and, 81–82
  (*See also* Drugs; *name of specific drug*)
Chlorambucil, 84

Choosing a wig (*see* Wigs)
Choroid, 115
Circles under eyes, 100
Circulation exercise, 210
cis-Platinum, 134
Clay mask, 102
Clergy, 230
Clip-on hairpiece, 49
Clothes after breast surgery, 154
   (*See also* Appearance)
Collagen, scars and, 90–91, 127, 152
Colostomy, 168
Commercial hair dye, 74
Communication, 223–224
Complex 15, 87, 103
Constipation, 177, 180–181
Contact lenses, 125
Control, feelings of, 227
Coping strategies, 216–217, 219–220
   positive denial in, 227–228
   state of readiness for change and, 12–13
Cornea, 115
Corporate Angel Network (CAN), 236
Cosmetics (*see* Makeup)
Cosmetological paramedics, 91
Cost:
   of breast prosthesis, 161–162
   of breast reconstruction, 164
   of counseling, 225
Counseling, 224–225
Covered heads, 63–72
Covermark camouflage makeup, 91
Creams:
   foundation, 99
   moisturizing, 86–87
Crew cuts, 26–29
Cryotherapy:
   oral cancer and, 143
   skin cancer around eye and, 117
Cure:
   involvement in treatment and, 221
   prediction of, 217–218
Custom-made wigs, 45–46
   (*See also* Wigs)
Cuticle, 129
Cyclophosphamide, 84
Cytosine arabinoside, 85

Dacarbazine, 89
D'Avray wigs, 54
Debulking, 10
DeMeo Brothers Hair, 238

Denial:
   hair loss and, 25
   positive, 227–228
Dentures, 138
Deodorant after breast surgery, 155–156
Depression:
   treatment for, 228–229
   weight gain and, 174
Dermablend camouflage makeup, 91
Dermal papilla, 18
Dermis, 81
Descending colostomy, 168
Diabetes, 134
Diary, 239
Diet, 173–183
   bloating and, 180–181
   calorie counting in, 180
   figure control in, 173–177
   food aversions in, 178–179
   mini-meals in, 177
   radiotherapy and, 176–177
   reasons for healthy, 178
   reducing, 175
   soft and simple, 181–183
   vitamins and, 179–180
Discoloration of tooth, 137–138
Diuretics, 180–181
Doctor, questions for, 220–223, 234
Dove cleansing bar, 102
Doxorubicin, 84
Drinking of alcoholic beverages, 142
Driving:
   buddy system and, 226
   limitations in, 156
Drugs:
   breast cancer and, 152
   for depression, 229
   hair and, 18–20
   skin and, 84–85
   (*See also* Chemotherapy; *name of specific drug*)
Dry eyes, 118–119
Dry lips, 139, 141–142
Dry mouth, 139–141
Dry skin, 83, 85–87

Eating habits, 178
Eczema, 85
Edith Imre wigs, 238
Eentsy weentsy spider exercise, 185–186
Elimination, ostomies and, 167–170
Emotions:
   breast surgery and, 153, 157

Emotions (*cont.*):
  cancer diagnosis and, 215–217
  gynecologic cancer and, 170
  mastectomy and, 153
  weight gain and, 174
  (*See also* Fears)
Encore, 236
Endocrine therapy, 152
Enemas, 181
Epidermis, 81
Erythema, 87
Eucerin, 86
Eva Gabor wigs, 47–48, 54, 238
Exercise, 183–213
  arm hoist, 208–209
  backward arm lift, 206–207
  eentsy weentsy spider, 185–186
  Gloria's rubber ball squeeze,
    188–189
  invisible-bear hug, 195–196
  leg, 210–213
  level of, 183
  little teapot, 192
  my lord, 193–194
  olympic gold, 204–206
  postmastectomy, 153–154, 183–209
    beginner, 185–199
    intermediate, 200–209
    weights in, 200–209
  pump two, 202–204
  Queen Elizabeth wave, 186–187
    modified, 201–202
  shoulder molders, 191
  stick 'em up, 211
  strenuous, 183
  swing low, 196–197
  swing low double O, 198–199
  walking as, 184
  warm-up for, 200
  wind in the willow, 189–190
Eye cancer, 116–118
Eye makeup, 96, 101, 104
  choosing, 100
  surgery and, 97
Eye mask, 125
Eyeball, cancer of, 117
Eyebrows, 119–126
  loss of makeup and, 101
  transplants of, 120
Eyelash curler, 100
Eyelashes, 119–126
  chemotherapy and, 100
  loss of makeup and, 101
  transfer of, 124

Eyes, 115–119
  cancer of, 116–118
  tricks for, 125–126

Fallout hair, 24–25
  (*See also* Hair loss)
False eyebrows, 120
False eyelashes, 121–123
Family support, 224, 225
Fatigue, exercise and, 183
Fears:
  of breast cancer, 146–147
  of breasts not growing, 146
  of hair loss, 20–21
  and talking it out, 223–224
Feelings (*see* Emotions)
Feet, 134
Fibrocystic breast, 147
Figure control, 173–177
Fingernails, 129–134
Fitness, baseline profile of, 8
  (*See also* Appearance)
5-Fluorouracil, 84, 88–89
Food:
  aversions to, 178–179
  as fuel, 178
  soft and simple, 181–183
  (*See also* Diet)
Food habits, 178
Foundation makeup, 99, 100
Fragrances, 96
Fred Hutchinson Cancer Research Center,
  236
Freezing:
  oral cancer and, 143
  skin cancer around eye and, 117
Frends Beauty Supply, 237
Fringes, 49

General Wig Company, 47
Getting better, 230–231
Getting help, 219–220
Getting information, 219–223, 234, 236–237
Glasses, 125–126
Globe, cancer of, 117
Gloria's rubber ball squeeze exercise, 188–189
Good looks (*see* Appearance)
Good Patient complex, 216, 220–221
Graft:
  eyelash, 124
  skin, 164, 166
Group counseling, 224–225

Gums, red or swollen, 139
Gynecologic surgery, 170–171

Hair, 15–35
    anatomy of, 18–19
    baseline profile of, 8
    color of, 75–77
    drugs and toxins and, 18–20
    growing back, 74–75
    loss of (*see* Hair loss)
    meaning of, 15–18
    pre-chemotherapy care of, 20–24
    pubic, 78–79
    Rapunzel syndrome and, 15–18
    thin, care of, 50–51
    virgin, 77–78
Hair color, 75–77
Hair loss:
    accepting, 26–28
    adjustment to, 33–35
    anticipation of, 20–24
    crew cuts and, 26–29
    denial of, 25
    fallout rate of, 24–25
    preparation for, 20–24
    prevention of, 31–33
    reactions to, 26–28, 33–35, 37–38
    types of, 29–31
Hair replacement (*see* Wigs)
Hair-saving techniques, hazards of, 33
Haircut before chemotherapy, 24–29
Hairdresser for crew cut, 27
Hairpieces, 49–50
Half-wigs, 49
Hand-tied wigs, 44–45
Hands, 128–129
Harvard pump, 9
Hats, 73–74
Head cancer, 127–128
Head coverings, 63–74
    (*See also* Wigs)
Henna, 74
Hodgkin's disease, 93
Hope, 4
Hormones after breast surgery, 155
Humidifier, 102
Humor, 5
Hydroxyurea, 84
Hyperpigmentation, 87–89
Hyperthermia, 10
Hypopigmentation, 88
Hypothermia, 31–33
Hysterectomy, 170

Ice cream, 177
Ice pack, 125
Ileostomy, 168
Imaging technique, 229
Immunotherapy, 11–12
Implants, radiation:
    breast, 151–152
    vaginal, 171
Individual counseling, 224–225
Infection:
    oral, 139
    prevention of, 155
Information, need for, 219–223, 234
Information groups, 236–237
Infusion device, 9, 33
    hair-saving techniques and, 33
    hyperpigmentation and, 88
Insurance:
    breast prosthesis and, 161–162
    counseling costs and, 225
    ostomy equipment and, 169
Interferon, 12
Invisible-bear hug exercise, 195–196
Iris, 115

Jacquelyn Wigs, 238
Jacques Darcel wigs, 238
Jones' Tube, 117

Keratin, 18, 129
Kimonos, 154
Knit cap, 63–70

Lacri-Lube, 119
Lacrisert, 119
LactiCare lotion, 86
Lancome mascara, 105
Laugh therapy, 5, 229
Laxatives, 181
Learning from other cancer patients, 222–223
Leg exercises, 210–213
Leukemia Society of America, 236
Lips, 141–142
Lipstick, 96, 97
Liquid-food products, 175–176
Little teapot exercise, 192
Looking good (*see* Appearance)
Loss of hair (*see* Hair loss)
Lotions, moisturizing, 86, 103
Lugo Hair Center, 238
Lumpectomy, 150, 151

Lumps in breast, 147
Lungs, 126–127
Lunula, 129

Mail-order wigs, 47–48
Make Today Count, 236
Makeup, 95–113
  benefits of, 5–7
  blush and, 105
  change in looks and, 113
  inpatient, 96–98
  makeovers in, 105–113
  outpatient, 98–103
  shopping list for, 232
  two-minute face, 103–105
  two-second blush, 105
Malignant melanoma, 93–94
Manicure, 130–132
  surgery and, 97
Mascara, 96, 101, 104–105
  choosing, 100, 105
  surgery and, 97
Mastectomy, 149–150
  adjustment to, 156–157
  alternatives to, 150–151
  breast prosthesis after (*see* Breast
    prosthesis)
  breast reconstruction after (*see* Breast
    reconstruction)
  exercises after, 153–154, 183–209
    beginning, 185–199
    intermediate, 200–209
  modified radical, 149
    reconstruction after, 163–164
  partial, 149–150
  preventive, 167
  radical, 149
    reconstruction after, 164
    recovery from, 152–156
  recovery from, 152–156
  simple, 149
  total, with axillary dissection, 149
  weight gain after, 174
Mechlorethamine, 84
Melanin, 88
Melanoma, malignant, 93–94
Methotrexate, 84–85, 89
Milk shakes, 175–177, 183
Mini-meals, 177
Minoxidil, 31
Mithramycin, 84
Modified radical mastectomy, 149
  reconstruction after, 163–164

Moisturizers, 85–87, 98, 99, 103
Moisturizing mask, 102
Moles, 93–94
Monoclonal antibodies, 12
Mouth, 138–141
  baseline profile of, 8
  cancer of, 142–143
  tenderness of, 139
My lord exercise, 193–194

Nail biters, 133–134
Nail polish, 97
Nails, 129–136
Natural Cover makeup, 91
Neck cancer, 127–128
Neutrogena, 86, 102
Nightgowns, 154
Nipple banking, 166
Nipples:
  breast prosthesis and, 159
  breast reconstruction and, 166
Nitrosoureas, 84
Nivea lotion, 86

Oat cell carcinoma of lung, 127
Olympic gold exercise, 204–206
Oral cancer, 142–143
Oral infections, 139
  (*See also* Mouth)
Ostomal Society, 169
Ostomies, 167–170
Ostomy equipment, 169
Ovarian cancer, 170

Padding for brassieres, 157–158
Pain of hair fallout, 25
Pain relief, 10
Painting of tooth, 137–138
Palliation, 10
Pancakes, 181–182
Paramedics, cosmetological, 91
Partial mastectomy, 149–150
Pasta, 179, 183
Patient buddy system, 225–226
Patient diary, 239
Patient involvement in treatment, 221–223
Pedicure, 135–136
Peel-off mask, 102
Perfumes, 96
Periods of adjustment, 217–218
Perms, 77

Personal resource list, 233
Petroleum jelly, 85–86
Phone number list, 233
Photoradiation, 11
Phototoxicity, 88–89
Pick, hair, 61
Pigment tattoo, 124
Pimples, scalp, 74
Plaque, dental, 139
Plastic surgery, oral, 143
cis-Platinum, 134
Pookey cap, 63–70
Positive denial, 227–228
Postmastectomy exercises, 153–154, 183–209
  beginning, 185–199
  intermediate, 200–209
  weights in, 200–209
Powder, makeup, 99–100
Prevention:
  hair loss, 31–33
  mastectomy for, 167
Prostheses, breast (*see* Breast prosthesis)
Prosthetics for Hair Loss, 238
  (*See also* Wigs)
Psychologists:
  breast surgery recovery and, 153, 157
  expression of real feelings and, 223
Pubic hair, loss of, 78–79
Pump two exercise, 202–204

Q-10 enzyme, 31
Quadrantectomy, 150
Queen Elizabeth wave exercise, 186–187
  modified, 201–202
Questions for doctor, 220–223, 234
Quick of nailbed, 129

Radiant irradiated skin, 89–90
Radiation:
  breast cancer and, 150–152
  complications of, 29–31, 83, 89
  in implants: for breast cancer, 151–152
    for vaginal cancer, 171
  skin cancer around eye and, 117
  (*See also* Radiotherapy)
Radiation burn, 83
Radiation implants, 151–152, 171
Radical mastectomy, 149
  modified, 149
    reconstruction after, 163–164
  reconstruction after, 164
  recovery from, 152–156

Radiodermatitis, 83
Radiotherapy, 10–11
  diet and, 176–177
  hair loss and, 29–31
  oral cancer and, 143
  secondary skin cancer and, 89
  skin and, 83–90
  (*See also* Radiation)
Rashes, 87
Reach for Recovery, 152, 236
Reactions, 3–4
  to hair loss, 26–28, 33–35, 37–38
  to wigs, 40–45
Recipes, 182–183
Reconstruction:
  breast (*see* Breast reconstruction)
  of vagina, 171
Recovery, 230–231
Red skin, 87
Reducing diet, 175
Regalia turbans, 237
Relaxation Response, The, 229
Relaxation training (ReT), 229
Religion, 230
René wigs, 47–48, 54–55, 238
Resource list, 233, 235
Responsibility for illness outcome, 226–227
ReT (relaxation training), 229
Retina, 115
Robes, 154
Rubber ball squeeze exercise, 153–154,
  188–189

Safety after breast surgery, 155
Saliva, decreased, 139–141
Scalp:
  pain and, 25
  pimples on, 74
Scalp cap, 32–33
Scars, 90–92
  from breast implants, 151–152
  from breast reconstruction, 164
  and collagen, 90–91, 127, 152
Sclera, 115
Segmentectomy, 150
Selective denial, 227–228
Self-pity, 216
Sense of humor, 5
Sexual pleasure, 171
Share, 236
Shopping:
  for breast prosthesis, 159–162
  for makeup, 232

Shopping (*cont.*):
　for wig, 23–24
Shoulder molders exercise, 191
Sigmoid colostomy, 168
Simple mastectomy, 149
Ski cap, 74
Skin, 81–95
　baseline profile of, 8
　cancer of, 92–94
　　eyes and, 116–117
　color of, 87–88
　dry, 85–87
　facts on, 81–82
　hyperpigmentation of, 87–88
　phototoxicity and, 88–89
　radiant irradiated, 89–90
　rashes of, 87
　red, 87
　scars of, 90–92
　　breast and, 151–152, 164
　sun care and (*see* Sunscreens)
　temporary versus permanent damage to,
　　89
　treatment effects on, 83–89
Skin cancer, 92–94
　eyes and, 116–117
Skin graft, 164, 166
Slink head cover, 71, 72
Small meals, 177
Smoking, 142
Snacks, series of, 177
Soap, 102
Societal attitudes, 218
Soft foods, 181–183
Sore feet, 134
Soups, 182, 183
SPF 15 sunscreen, 95, 99, 103, 156
Squamous cell carcinoma, 93
　eyes and, 116–117
　of lung, 127
Squeezing exercise, 153–154,
　　188–189
Stick 'em up exercise, 211
Stoma, 167
Stomatitis, 139
Styles, wig, 38–40, 54–55, 58–60
Subclavian lines, 9
Sun:
　phototoxicity and, 88–89
　skin cancer and, 93
　skin care and, 95, 99, 103, 156
Sun block, 95
Sunburn, 156
Sunscreens, 95, 99, 103, 156

Support, 224–225
　from other cancer patients, 222–223
Support groups:
　breast surgery and, 157
　list of, 236–237
Survival, desire for, 4
Suzy's Blend, 103
Swallowing, difficulty in, 139
Swelling, 134, 180–181
Swing low double O exercise, 198–199
Swing low exercise, 196–197
Swollen ankles, 134
Swollen face, 181
Synthetic wigs, 44–45
　lifespan of, 56
　(*See also* Wigs)

Taking responsibility for illness outcome,
　　226–227
Talking it out, 223–224
Tattoo, pigment, 124
Teeth, 136–138
Theatrical eyebrows, 120
Therapy (*see* Treatment)
Thin-hair tricks, 50–51
Three-quarter wig, 49
Toenails, 134–136
Tongue, 139
Total mastectomy with axillary dissection,
　　149
Toupee tape, 61
Tracheostomy, 128
Transition, 113
Transplants or transfer:
　eyebrow, 120
　eyelash, 124
Transverse colostomy, 168
Treatment:
　antidepression, 228–229
　patient involvement in, 221–223
　skin and, 83–89
　(*See also* Cancer treatment; *specific cancer and
　　specific treatment*)
Turbans, 70, 237
Tuttle theatrical makeup, 91
Two-minute face makeup, 103–105

United Cancer Council, 236
United Ostomy Association, 237
Urinary diversion, 168
Urostomy, 168
Uterine cancer, 170

Vagina, reconstruction of, 171
Vaseline, 85–86
Veneer, tooth, 138
Vinblastine, 89
Vincristine, 134
Virgin hair, 77–78
Visualization technique, 229
Vital Options, 237
Vitamins, 179–180
Vulva, cancer of, 170

Walking, 184
Warm-up for exercise, 200
Washing:
  and bathing, 85
  of hair, 50, 77
  of wigs, 60
Water-based makeup, 99
Water retention, 180–181
Watteau, Jean-Antoine, 71, 72
Weight gain, 173, 174
  chemotherapy and, 174–175
  reducing diet and, 175
Weight loss, 173–174
  diet supplements and, 175–176
Weights for exercise, 200–209
Wet reaction of skin, 83
White plaque, 139
Why Me syndrome, 3–4, 216
  weight gain and, 174
Wig brush, 61

Wig makers, 45–46
Wigless possibilities, 61–62
Wigs, 37–61
  beginner, 23–24, 51–54
  care of, 60–61
  choosing, 57–59
  color of, 39–40, 58
  custom-made, 45–46
  fashion, 53
  hairpieces and, 49–50
  human-hair, 44–45
  lifespan of, 56
  makeup and, 102–103
  multiple, 55–57
  reactions to, 40–45
  ready-to-wear, 46–48
  rip-offs in, 48
  shopping for, 23–24
  styles of, 38–40, 54–55, 58–60
  suppliers of, 237–238
  supplies for, 61
  thin-hair tricks and, 50–51
  tricks for, 38–40
Wigs of France, 47–48, 54
Wind in the willow exercise, 189–190
Wounds, chemotherapy and, 81–82
Wrinkles, 102

Xerosis, 85
X-rays, 10
  (*See also* Radiation; Radiotherapy)